The Biological Basis of Nursing: Clinical Observations

A thorough understanding of the biological science underlying fundamental nursing observations such as taking the temperature or measuring the pulse enables nurses to make well-informed clinical decisions quickly and accurately.

The Biological Basis of Nursing: Clinical Observations integrates clear explanations of the techniques involved in these procedures with the biological knowledge which gives them meaning. For each topic, William Blows explains the pathological basis for variations in observed results. This helpful text gives nurse practitioners at all levels the understanding needed to:

- perform clinical observations accurately
- make accurate judgements about the patient's condition
- make accurate decisions concerning patient care

It looks at:

- temperature
- cardiovascular observations (the pulse and blood pressure)
- respiratory observations
- eliminatory observations (urinary and digestive)
- neurological observations (consciousness, eyes, movement)

The basic observations taught at the start of training are explored at a fundamental level, while neurological observations are explained in more depth. Generously illustrated, this is an essential text for nurses in training. It will also be of great use to clinical staff and nurse educators.

William T. Blows is a lecturer in Applied Biological Sciences at St Bartholomew College of Nursing, City University, London.

The Biological
Basis of Nursing:
Clinical Observations

William T. Blows

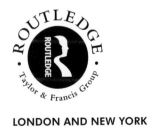

LONDON AND NEW YORK

First published 2001
by Routledge
11 New Fetter Lane, London EC4P 4EE

Simultaneously published in the USA and
Canada
by Routledge
29 West 35th Street, New York, NY 10001

*Routledge is an imprint of the Taylor & Francis
Group*

© 2001 William T. Blows

Typeset in Janson and Futura by Prepress
Projects Ltd, Perth, Scotland

Printed and bound in Great Britain by
TJ International Ltd, Padstow, Cornwall

British Library Cataloguing in Publication Data
A catalogue record for this book is available
from the British Library

*Library of Congress Cataloging-in-Publication
Data*
Blows, William T., 1947–
　The biological basis of nursing: clinical
　observations/William T. Blows
　　　p. cm.
　Includes bibliographical references.
　1. Nursing. 2. Clinical medicine. 3.
　Biology. 4. Human physiology. I. title.
　[DNLM: 1. Clinical Medicine – Nurses'
　Instruction. 2. Physiological Processes –
　Nurses' Instruction. 3. Decision Making –
　Nurses' Instruction. QT 104 B657b 2000]
　RT42.B576 2000
　610.73–dc21　00-032355
　CIP
　ISBN 0–415–21254–5 (hbk.) –
　ISBN 0-415-21255-3 (pbk.)

Contents

Figures

Tables

Preface

Biological sciences in nursing has seen a change in status over the last 20 years. As a nurse educator, I became aware that with the introduction of the 'nursing model' all signs of biology were banished from the curriculum. Anatomy and physiology were thought to be akin to the 'medical model', and as such they fell outside the nurse's territory. At all costs, nurses had to be seen as autonomous practitioners in their own right. But autonomy at what price? Several generations of nurses were trained with minimal understanding of how the body works, or how it reacts to trauma, drugs and disease. They had little conception of how the body responded to the nurse's own interventions. One surgical consultant angrily telephoned the School of Nursing to say that a third year student nurse did not even know where the liver was. It is a legacy that the profession is still suffering from.

Fortunately, today more nurses than ever are taking biological studies seriously, from diploma to masters level, and as autonomous practitioners they have discovered, more than ever, that the sciences are vital to their work. They understand that their client has a problem affecting a physiological system, and the treatment, something they are an integral part of, has a biological focus, often in the form of drugs or surgery. Nurses today, as clinical specialists, are taking on more advanced work, often in areas previously thought of as being in the domain of the doctor. These nurses need to be taught skills during the first weeks of training which are themselves based on sound knowledge. One of the skills they need is clinical decision-making, often carried out quickly and under pressure. A thorough understanding of the underpinning sciences is essential to broaden the number of choices available and to facilitate making the correct choice.

In addition, medical sciences have never seen such a remarkable flood of new knowledge as we are seeing today; knowledge that will revolutionise the way we treat disease. Advances in genetics and neuroscience are two good examples of this. If nurses are going to remain at the 'coal face' of this revolution, they must be conversant with the sciences and technologies that underpin the changing face of the care they give.

This book takes one of the most important care activities carried out by all nurses, the main clinical observations, and explores the biology behind them, giving the pathological basis for variations in the observed results. The basic observations usually taught at the start of the training programme are explored at a fundamental level, whereas neurological observations, often taught later in the curriculum and important for the specialist nurse, are a little more advanced.

This book will be of use and interest not only to students but also to nurse teachers and clinical staff.

William T. Blows

Chapter 1

Temperature

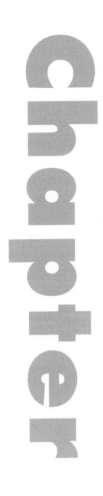

- Introduction
- Heat gain
- Heat movement and loss
- Heat regulation: gain versus loss
- Temperature scales and normal temperature variation
- Taking the body temperature in adults
- Taking the body temperature in children
- Abnormal high body temperatures
- Abnormal cold body temperatures
- Thermal injury
- Key points

Introduction

A great deal of mechanism exists within the body in order to stabilise the internal environment, and this is particularly important with regards to body temperature. At 37°C the human temperature is well balanced to provide the optimum conditions for tissue metabolism. Cooler temperatures would slow down the rate of cellular chemistry, which in turn would reduce cellular function. As it is, most chemical changes require enzymes to speed up the reactions to a level necessary for life. When these temperature-sensitive reactions are cooled, the resultant slowing of metabolism becomes dangerous to health. Hotter temperatures are also problematic, by causing metabolic systems to become inefficient and enzymes to move closer to denaturing. **Denaturing** is a heat-related change in protein structure which again creates failure of cellular activity.

This essential stabilisation of optimum temperatures must happen despite changes in the external environmental temperature (known as the **ambient temperature**). It is only with help from external factors such as clothes and fires that humans can survive in temperatures that may otherwise be hostile to their cellular chemistry. Survival in the tropics or at the poles is entirely dependent on the body's ability to stabilise the internal environment aided by behaviour designed to retain or lose heat. But extremes of external temperature put great pressures on the body's systems, and they may fail to cope. The resulting dangerous change in a person's internal temperature is the cause of many deaths in very hot or very cold countries, or during very hot or very cold periods occurring in a usually temperate climate.

Measurement of body temperature becomes important for two reasons: it gives insight into the metabolic and homeostatic activity of the body and may also provide information about the possible cause of any abnormal state, contributing to an accurate diagnosis. For the body to balance the temperature, mechanisms must be in place to ensure that the heat gained is equal to the heat lost.

Heat gain

Heat production is part of the energy obtained from the use of the high-energy molecule **ATP (adenosine triphosphate)** in cellular metabolism. All cells use ATP, but some use more than others (e.g. liver and muscle cells) and therefore they liberate more heat. ATP itself is constructed from **ADP (adenosine diphosphate)** using energy from nutrients in the diet. Enzymes within the **mitochondrion**, an organelle at the centre of cellular respiration (i.e. the powerhouse of the cell), produce ATP from the metabolism of glucose and fat.

Glucose

Glucose is the end product of dietary carbohydrate breakdown by the digestive tract and the liver. One gram of glucose can be used by the body to produce about 4 kilocalories of energy, and this is known as the **Atwater number** for glucose. Glucose undergoes glycolysis in the cytoplasm close to the mitochondria. **Glycolysis** is the breakdown of glucose to the substance pyruvate, which can enter the mitochondrial matrix and join the **tricarboxylic** (or **Krebs**) **cycle**. Pyruvate will first become **acetyl-CoA** (**acetyl coenzyme A**), the entry point for substances joining the cycle. Throughout the cycle a series of reactions occurs which results in a return to acetyl-CoA (see Figure 1.1). The purpose of this cycle is twofold. First, it is a means of shedding excess carbon by combining it with oxygen (O_2) to form the waste gas carbon dioxide (CO_2). Second, it produces hydrogen (H) atoms that are transported to a chain reaction series, the **electron transport system**. The molecules moving the hydrogen from the Krebs cycle to the electron transport system on the inner mitochondrial membrane are **NAD** (**nicotinamide adenine dinucleotide**) and **FAD** (**flavine adenine dinucleotide**), which bind to the hydrogen to form **NADH** and **FADH$_2$** respectively. The hydrogen atoms, at the point of delivery to the first component of the electron transport chain, are split into **ions**, i.e. particles having a positive or negative charge, in this case protons (H^+) and the electrons (e^-). The protons are pumped out of the matrix to a position between the inner and outer mitochondrial membranes, and the electrons are passed down the electron transport system (Figure 1.2). Using enzymes bound to the inner-membrane folds (known as **cristae**) of the mitochondrion (Figure 1.3), this transport system releases electron energy in stages and immediately locks it up by the conversion of ADP and inorganic phosphate (P_i) to ATP. This generates some heat, but more heat will be liberated later when the ATP is used by the cell for other activities (i.e. the ATP is reduced again to ADP and P_i). Heat is then available for contribution to body temperature. The hydrogen ions that had been previously pumped out return to the matrix, an energy-liberating process driving the enzyme ATPase to further convert ADP and P_i to ATP, and thus store more

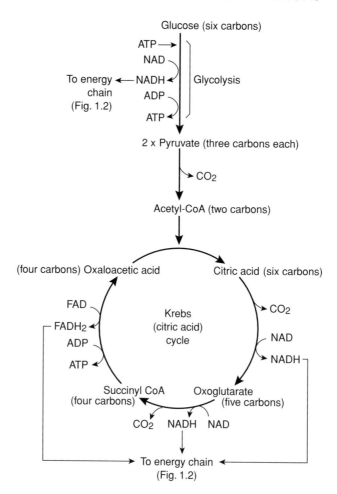

FIGURE 1.1 The Krebs (citric acid, tricarboxylic acid) cycle. Two pyruvates are obtained for each glucose as a result of glycolysis. Some ATP is needed to start the process. From pyruvate, acetyl coenzyme A (CoA) feeds into the cycle by binding to oxaloacetic acid to form citric acid. The carbon count of each step is shown, and at various points carbon is lost by combining with oxygen to form CO_2. NAD (nicotinamide adenine dinucleotide) and FAD (flavine adenine dinucleotide) combine with hydrogen at the points shown to transport this energy-rich hydrogen to the energy chain (Figure 1.2). ADP (adenosine diphosphate) becomes energy-rich ATP (adenosine triphosphate) during glycolysis and the cycle.

energy. The reunion of the electron and proton to form hydrogen again at the end of the process is accompanied by the further introduction of oxygen to create water ($2H^+ + 2e^- \rightarrow 2H + O \rightarrow H_2O$).

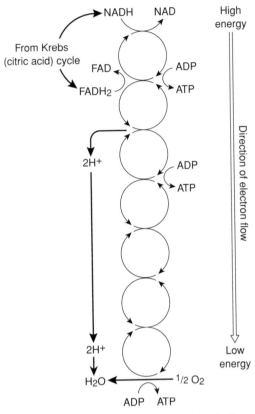

Figure 1.2 Electron transport chain. A simplified diagram of the cyclic reactions that electrons pass down from the high-energy end to the low-energy end. Hydrogen ions (H$^+$) and electrons arrive from the Krebs cycle transported by nicotinamide adenine dinucleotide (NAD) and flavine adenine dinucleotide (FAD). As the electrons flow down the chain reactions they lose energy, which is used to convert adenosine diphosphate (ADP) to adenosine triphosphate (ATP). The hydrogen ions pass directly to the end of the chain reaction where they join oxygen (half of O$_2$) to form metabolic water (H$_2$O). This takes place on the inner membrane cristae of the mitochondrion.

Fats

Whereas glucose enters the Krebs cycle via pyruvate, fats provide energy somewhat differently. The Atwater number for fats is about 9 kilocalories per 1 g, more than twice that of glucose. Fats occur in the diet as **triglycerides**, that is three (tri-) fatty acids attached to a single glycerol molecule. The molecule takes on a letter E shape (Figure 1.4). Fatty acids can be split from the glycerol by the enzyme **lipase**, and free glycerol can be converted to glucose by the liver, a process called **gluconeogenesis** (i.e. genesis = creation, neo = new; the creation

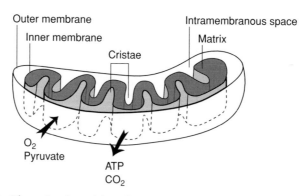

FIGURE 1.3 The mitochondrion. Pyruvate enters the matrix from the outside where glycolysis takes place. The matrix is the site of the Krebs cycle. The energy transport chain occurs on the cristae of the inner membrane. Oxygen (O_2) enters and combines with carbon to form carbon dioxide (CO_2). Adenosine triphosphate (ATP) leaves and passes to all parts of the cell.

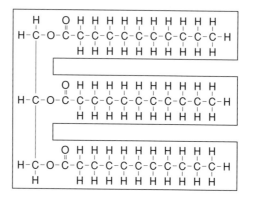

FIGURE 1.4 The E-shaped triglyceride molecule. A glycerol backbone holds together three long carbon (C) chain fatty acids saturated with hydrogen (H) and some oxygen (O).

of new glucose, or creating glucose from a non-carbohydrate source, as in this case from fats). This new glucose can be used by the liver and the rest of the body in the same way as glucose from carbohydrate. Free fatty acids from the triglyceride molecule can be used by the liver for the Krebs cycle, but they do not form pyruvate first. Instead, they enter the cycle by converting to acetyl-CoA and carrying on around the cycle from there. Thus, fatty acids provide an alternative, more direct input into the cycle other than via pyruvate (Figure 1.5). Fatty acids arriving at the liver in too large a quantity, as in **diabetes**, cannot

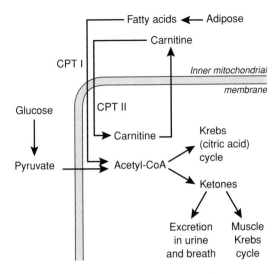

FIGURE 1.5 The entry of fatty acids into the Krebs citric acid cycle is an alternative pathway to glucose as an energy source. Movement of fatty acids across the inner mitochondrial membrane is effected by binding with carnitine, which is recycled. Binding with carnitine requires one form of the enzyme carnitine palmitoyltransferase I (CPT I), and removal of carnitine requires the other form CPT II. Some acetyl-CoA goes on to become ketones, which can be used for muscle energy or excreted.

all become acetyl-CoA, so they go through a different process leading to **ketone** formation, mostly **acetone**, which is excreted in the urine or breath, having been taken first via the blood to the kidneys or lungs. Normally, muscles are capable of taking up ketones from the blood for use as energy, including heat, but in diabetes this use of ketones may be blocked.

Proteins

Proteins, the body's vital nitrogen source, can also be used for heat production if absolutely necessary. Normally, carbohydrates are the first source of energy, followed by fats if carbohydrates are not available in the diet (e.g. in the case of starvation) or cannot be used by the body (e.g. in the case of diabetes). If fats are not available either (e.g. because of depletion of stored adipose) protein will be used as a last resort. Whereas fats used for energy causes weight loss, protein used for energy causes **muscle wasting**, and usually this means that the patient is in a very serious state of ill-health. Muscle wasting is mostly seen in patients who are dying from a terminal disease, such as cancer, and this state, called **cachexia**, results in debility, weakness, emaciation and a mental state of hopelessness. In order to use **amino acids** from proteins as an energy source, the liver must first remove the nitrogenous component, the amine group, a process called **deamination** (Figure 1.6), and convert the rest to glucose (gluconeogenesis again, this time glucose from protein). This glucose can be used as blood sugar to provide energy for cells, giving protein the same Atwater number as carbohydrates, 4 kilocalories per gram. The nitrogen within the amine group becomes **ammonia (NH$_3$)**, but small quantities only may be released from the liver into the blood since ammonia is toxic and should not be distributed widely in large amounts. Most of the ammonia is further converted in the liver to **urea** via the **Krebs urea cycle**. Urea is a safer compound to enter the blood and excrete through the kidneys and skin, but it can be toxic if blood levels are constantly raised.

Metabolism

Since **metabolism** is the total of all the chemical reactions in the body that use energy, and therefore liberate heat, it follows that there is a

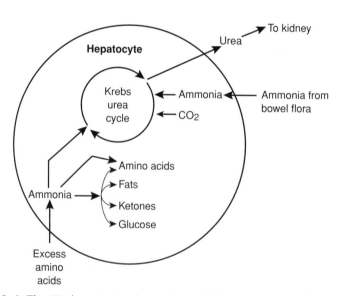

FIGURE 1.6 The Krebs urea cycle in liver cell (hepatocytes). Excess amino acids are split to release ammonia (NH$_3$). The remaining component can then be converted to glucose, fats or ketones. Some may join with ammonia to form amino acids again. Ammonia from bowel flora joins the cycle with CO$_2$ to form urea for excretion.

minimum rate of metabolism below which cellular activity may fail, with a subsequent threat to life. Overall, the **basal metabolic rate (BMR)** refers to the minimum total internal energy expenditure when awake but at rest, or the minimum metabolic rate at rest needed to sustain life. As would be expected, more heat energy is produced in areas of the body where cells exist that undergo high metabolic rates (e.g. the liver, but also the brain when active) or undertake movement (e.g. the muscles during exercise). The common factor between these areas is the rapid release of energy, creating heat as an excess product. The body creates an average of about 420 kilojoules (100 calories) of heat per hour, which would raise the body temperature by 2°C per hour if it were not lost at a rate equal to that at which it is produced (Blows 1998). Cells rich in mitochondria are clearly candidates for rapid metabolic rates and therefore high heat production. Areas of the body that house the greater number of cells away from the surface, i.e. the body core (notably the trunk, not the limbs) are sites where heat cannot escape directly into the environment, and are therefore hotter (Figure 1.7). They would be much hotter if heat was not moved away from the core by the blood.

Heat movement and loss

About 1°C difference exists between the **core temperature** and the **peripheral temperature**, but this difference can increase in cold environments to the extent that the hands and feet can be as much as 10°C cooler than the trunk (Figure 1.7). As more heat is produced it is essential that heat is moved away from the hotter core to the cooler surface tissues by the blood, the main transport system of the body. This is a major role of blood that is often overlooked. Moving heat in this manner is crucial to prevent very active tissues, such as the brain and liver, from overheating and virtually cooking themselves *in situ*. At the same time, tissues in direct contact with the external environment, the skin and mucous membranes, will not produce enough heat in extreme cold conditions to survive and rely entirely on heat transported into the tissues by the blood.

Removal of heat from the body is achieved mostly through the skin. Some heat is lost in faeces and urine, and in exhaled air, since inhaled air is warmed by the nasal and respiratory passages. Sweating is a very important means of heat loss and is a key indicator that the body is too hot. About two million sweat glands exist in a single individual, with

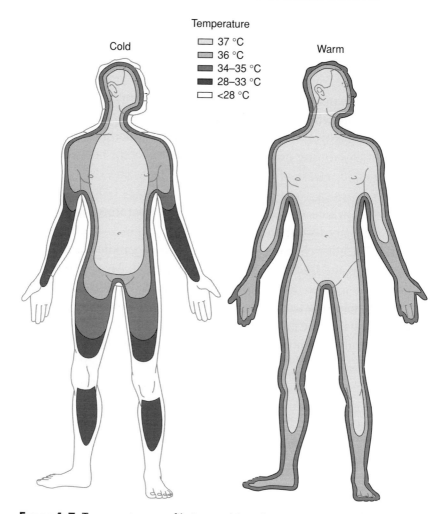

FIGURE 1.7 Temperature profile in a cold and in a warm environment. Notice the restricted core temperature (37°C) in the cold environment, keeping vital organs warm while minimising heat loss from the extremities. Under these conditions, the temperature of the extremities can be as much as 10°C lower than the core.

greater concentrations in specific areas like the axilla and palms. Excessive body heat is used to convert the sweat from a liquid state to a vapour. The heat used for this purpose is not registered as a temperature increase in the sweat, therefore it is called the **latent heat**, or hidden heat of evaporation. Sweat vapour then passes into the air taking this heat with it. In high-temperature situations, like a hot day or a high body temperature (e.g. infections or excessive exercise), sweating becomes a vital means of cooling the skin, which can then accept more heat from the core. An environment of high humidity severely reduces the skin's ability to vaporise sweat, and as the skin temperature rises so does the core.

Other means of skin heat loss are conduction, convection and radiation. Conduction is the passage of heat from the skin into any cooler object touching it. We warm the bed we sleep in, the clothes we wear, the seats we sit on, the pens we hold, and so on, by conduction. It is all heat lost from our cells. However, it constitutes the smallest amount of heat lost during the day unless the body is suddenly immersed in cold water, when rapid conduction can cause quick and severe hypothermia. Convection involves the warming of air next to the skin. Since warm air rises, it moves upwards and is replaced by colder air from below. The process is repeated continuously, making humans mobile convector heaters warming any environment they inhabit. This warm air layer is rapidly removed by wind, and if this wind is cold it causes the body to chill quickly, a phenomenon known as **the wind chill factor**. Radiation of heat is also continuous, where heat passes directly out from the skin into any objects it hits, warming that object. Gas or electric fires heat a room in the same way. By this means humans warm the walls, floors, ceilings and objects in a room. It is this form of heat that is picked up by thermal imaging cameras used in rescues from earthquake-damaged buildings and in night vision. With all these mechanisms of heat loss, it is not surprising that a class of students will themselves gradually raise the temperature of a cold classroom!

Heat regulation: gain versus loss

The body must have the ability to switch from increased heat production when it is cold to increased heat loss when it is hot. This is a finely tuned process that is sensitive to small changes in both the internal and the external temperature. Like any homeostatic mechanism, the aim is to stabilise the normal state, often called **normothermia**; in this case to sustain an average 37°C and to try to distribute heat evenly to all the tissues. Like any homeostatic mechanism, it involves sensory feedback to the brain and an output to effector organs. It is a negative feedback mechanism in which the system changes the direction of the original stimulus, i.e. if the temperature goes up the mechanism drives it down, and vice versa.

The area of the brain responsible for this control of temperature is the **hypothalamus**, the body's thermostat. The **preoptic nucleus** of the hypothalamus is rich in both heat- and cold-sensitive neurones able to monitor the temperature of the blood that passes through it and initiates any necessary maintenance action. The heat-sensitive neurones fire impulses faster as temperature rises, with a similar response from the cold-sensitive neurones to cooler temperatures (Guyton and Hall 1996). Peripheral and ambient temperatures are also monitored by both cold- and heat-sensitive receptors in the skin, and internal temperatures are monitored by sensors within the spinal cord, the abdominal organs and around the major veins. In all these areas cold receptors dominate, indicating the need for the body to avoid low rather than high temperatures. They feed back to the hypothalamus, the brain area that therefore has complete second-by-second information on the total body temperature (Guyton and Hall 1996). The hypothalamus maintains a **set point** of 37.1°C and initiates any changes necessary to stabilise the temperature at this set point. Any situation that causes the body temperature to rise above the set point (i.e. **hyperthermia**, **pyrexia** or **hyperpyrexia**) results in the hypothalamus activating the **sympathetic nervous system**, which stimulates sweating. At the same time, *reduced* sympathetic **vasoconstrictor tone** causes vasodilatation of the skin vessels coupled with relaxation of the precapillary sphincters. Together these ensure more blood brings more heat to the body surface, causing the skin to be hot and flushed. Skin blood flow can vary from 250 ml to as much as 2,500 ml per minute depending on thermoregulatory needs (Watson 1998). Sympathetic stimulation also results in an associated increase in heart rate, ensuring faster delivery of blood to the skin, and an increase in the respiratory rate. Behavioural changes also occur; the individual removes clothes or bedding to get comfortable and takes a cold drink or cooling shower.

In **hypothermia** (body temperature below the set point, i.e. 35°C or lower) the hypothalamus initiates sympathetic activity that increases cellular metabolism to generate more heat, and it *increases* sympathetic **vasoconstrictor tone**, which will constrict the peripheral blood vessels in the skin to reduce the heat loss. Sweating is shut down and respirations are reduced. It may seem contradictory that the sympathetic nervous system can be activated in both extremes of body temperature and yet have different effects. This is because the sympathetic nervous system uses the neurotransmitter **noradrenaline** at the termination synapse, and this binds to different receptors with varying results. Hair erector (or pilomotor) muscles cause hairs to stand on end, a process that should trap more air next to the skin for improved insulation. Its use is probably limited in humans due to the sparseness of hair compared with animals and the wearing of clothing. It does, however, cause the goose pimples that clearly indicate that the skin is chilled. The **motor nervous system** supplying the skeletal muscle is used to increase muscle tone in a manner that induces shivering, again to boost heat production, as all muscle activity does. The motor system also enhances conscious behavioural responses, like turning on heating systems, exercise and dressing warmly.

Temperature scales and normal temperature variation

The body temperature is measured in degrees Celsius (or **centigrade**, °C) as part of the **Standard International (SI) system**. Strictly speaking, the SI unit for temperature is the **Kelvin (K)**, but this is rather impractical for clinical use since 0 K is *minus* 273 degrees centigrade (–273°C, i.e. the lowest, or coldest, known temperature), making body temperature 310 K. Centigrade uses 0°C as the freezing point of water and 100°C as the boiling point of water at one atmosphere air pressure (generally accepted as sea level). This last point is important since boiling point is dependent on the air pressure and water boils at reduced temperatures as air pressure drops, i.e. when ascending away from sea level. In outer space, for example, the freezing and boiling points of water meet: water would instantly freeze due to the very low temperatures and, at the same time, boil due to zero air pressure! The centigrade scale has taken over from the **Fahrenheit** (°F) system, which had the freezing point at 32°F and the boiling point at 212°F. The body temperature at 37°C was previously measured at 98.4°F, a figure which may still be found in older texts. The conversion of Centigrade to Fahrenheit uses the formula 1.8 (°C) + 32 = °F, i.e. taking the normal body temperature of 37 °C as an example, 1.8 × 37 = 66.6; then 66.6 + 32 = 98.6 °F (Figure 1.8).

Normally small local changes in peripheral body temperature are to be expected as a result of variations in the external air temperature or contact with hot or cold surfaces. Such circumstances arise in very hot or very cold weather and in work environments that involve molten metal or refrigeration. These variations can cause thermal injuries if over exposure occurs. A normal diurnal (24-hour) pattern of fluctuations also occurs, with lowest temperatures in the morning and highest in the evening. The body is also hotter after a warm bath or shower, and

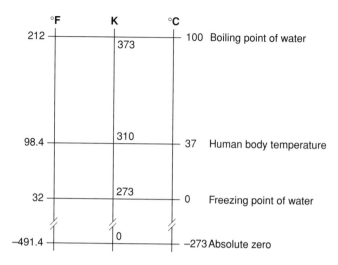

Figure 1.8 The Kelvin, Celsius (centigrade) and Fahrenheit temperature scales. The correlation between absolute 0, the freezing point of water, the human body temperature and the boiling point of water is shown.

the core temperature will be temporarily increased by a hot drink, making oral measurement deceptive.

Taking the body temperature in adults

The traditional means of taking the temperature, i.e. the oral route, is still useful as it measures the temperature of the blood in the carotid artery, blood that is coming directly from the core temperature (Watson 1998). The peripheral and core temperatures are different because the peripheral temperature has the role of losing heat and therefore can fluctuate with the ambient temperature state. The core temperature must remain constant and is therefore the most accurate temperature to measure. It is the only stable temperature available, and it is also the temperature at which the vital organs must exist and function. Other routes such as the axilla, groin, rectum and ear are used, especially in specific client groups or certain situations when oral temperatures are inappropriate. The elderly, the mentally disturbed and very young children are groups where the oral route is likely to be inadvisable.

The clinical thermometer has now largely been replaced by electronic probes, partly because of the risks associated with breakage of glass and mercury toxicity, and partly to resolve the problems of the time needed for accuracy. O'Toole (1998) gives a good overall assessment of the sites and methods for taking the body temperature. She identified four types of thermometer as mercury-in-glass, disposable, electronic and infrared; all of which are in clinical use.

Mercury thermometers have been in use for a long time and are recognised as reasonably accurate (if left in place long enough, usually at least 3 minutes see p. 16) and convenient. Several variations are known, including the normal and low scale range oral versions, and the rectal versions with a blue bulb or a blue dot. A restriction in the mercury (Hg) column traps the mercury in the column and allows the temperature to be read outside the body without the mercury contracting back to the bulb. However, preparation for repeated use requires careful shaking of the instrument to force the mercury back into the bulb. This is when most breakages occur, with the double hazard of broken glass and released mercury. Mercury is now recognised as a toxic hazard, especially if inhaled as vapour, which can remain in the environment for months after mercury spillage from a glass thermometer. Skin and mucous membrane absorption of mercury is poor, but the vapour is well absorbed through the lungs. Removal of spilt mercury via a vacuum cleaner is not recommended as this vaporises the metal and sprays the vapour around the house (Anon. 1996). In 1995, a total of 622 calls were made to the National Poisons Information Service about mercury poisoning, mostly concerning broken thermometers, and the majority of these breakages happened in the home (Anon. 1996). Acute mercury poisoning (within 30 minutes) results in thirst, nausea, vomiting, abdominal pains, diarrhoea with blood and ultimately renal failure. Chronic mercury toxicity involves irritability, excessive salivation, loose teeth, gum disorders, slurred speech, tremors and unsteady gait. Broken glass causes additional risks with mercury thermometer accidents, e.g. rectal perforations, oral injury and swallowed glass fragments. These problems limit the use of the traditional clinical thermometer, and it will ultimately be replaced in most clinical areas by one of the other types. Special guidelines and mercury spillage kits are available for dealing with thermometer breakages, and these should be at hand for such events, with staff trained in this procedure. Cross-infection by glass thermometers is another problem that has never been fully resolved, as disinfection is not always convenient, desirable or effective, and disposable plastic covers, called dispotemps, can sometimes break. Organic matter left behind on thermometers after use, house and grow a variety of organisms including the influenza virus and *Clostridium* (Anon. 1996). The problem of accuracy in temperature measurement in glass thermometers has been discussed in the literature for a long time, with the focus on how long to leave the instrument in place. Three minutes has been the usual practice, but studies have identified longer time spans, sometimes up to 9 minutes, to achieve full accuracy. This length of time is of course impractical and unwarranted on a busy ward. Studies have shown that a difference of only 0.1°C exists between 3 and 9 minutes. Given these problems, it is not surprising that with modern technology the mercury-in-glass thermometer is destined to become a museum piece.

Disposable thermometers are now available and are as accurate as mercury and electronic thermometers. They are each about one-tenth of the price of the traditional mercury thermometer (O'Toole 1998) but are for single use only. A series of temperature-sensitive chemical colour change dots provides an easily read system. Erickson *et al.* (1996) identified variations in temperature with these chemical-dot skin-recording methods when compared with electronic devices in the same site (oral and axilla) in adults and children. Differences of ±0.4°C occurred frequently, suggesting that skin devices of this kind only allow an approximation of the body temperature (i.e. they record peripheral temperatures).

Electronic devices are available for oral, axillary and rectal use. They take just 1 or 2 minutes to achieve a result in most cases, which is beneficial to both the busy nurse and the patient. Accuracy is generally on a par with the mercury thermometer in standard ward situations (O'Toole 1998).

Infrared thermometers are primarily for use in the ear, measuring the temperature of the tympanic membrane quickly, sometimes in seconds (Anon. 1996). This route is now of growing importance, and it has been recognised that the ear drum shares the same blood supply as the hypothalamus, which makes it very close to core temperature, equating well with pulmonary artery temperature in some studies (O'Toole 1998). It is also easily accessible with a short probe, similar to those on an otoscope, that fits into the external canal of the ear. The lens on the tip of the probe must face the membrane and a good seal should be obtained around the probe to ensure that only body heat is sampled. The presence of cerumen (ear wax) may give a reading lower than reality. This method has been used on sleeping patients without waking them. The infrared probe is probably better used on adults and older children, who not only have reasonably formed external ear canals (see p. 17) but will co-operate better with the procedure.

Taking the body temperature in children

There has been a considerable debate in the literature about the route for taking temperatures in children. Some sources suggest that the rectal route, chosen because very young children cannot comply with the oral route and it was more accurate than the axillary route, was dangerous because of the risk of rectal perforation and other complications. However, Morley (1992) identified multiple reasons for choosing rectal temperature measurements in infants and young children rather than the axillary route, and presented evidence to show the inaccuracy of axillary measurements in the very young. The difference between axillary and rectal temperatures in children can be as much as 3°C, and axillary measurements would miss one-quarter of febrile babies (Morley *et al.* 1992). Shape changes in the external canal as a result of different growth stages in children may affect the use of the infrared probe and therefore the accuracy of this type of thermometer. This may be one reason why tympanic measurements of temperature have been reported not to have registered a fever in some children and are probably inappropriate in neonates (Davis 1993). A special infrared probe is designed and available for axillary use in neonates. Currently, the ideal method of clinical temperature taking in small children appears to be via the rectal route, but not everyone is convinced of this and the debate continues.

Abnormal high body temperatures

Fevers are high temperatures, i.e. above 38°C (Blumenthal 1998); a **pyrexia** is recognised as a continuous body temperature above 37.5°C up to 39.9°C, and a hyperpyrexia is 40°C or above (Harker and Gibson 1995). Raised temperatures are caused by toxins or drug reactions, infections, prolonged exposure to a hot environment, brain disorders affecting the hypothalamus, neoplasms, autoimmune diseases or the penguin effect (Blows 1998) (see p. 18). Under any of these circumstances the body may fail to control the temperature by the means identified earlier, notably sweating, when the set point (see p. 12) is exceeded. The hypothalamic set point is the role of the preoptic nucleus, and it is largely influenced by feedback from the peripheral skin, spinal cord and abdominal visceral temperatures. However, in fevers, first the hypothalamic set point is driven up to a higher level, e.g. 39°C, in a regulated manner, unlike in hyperthermia in which there is an unregulated temperature rise (Henker *et al.* 1997). In fever, the control centre perceives normal temperature as being too low. Heat conservation and heat production then drive the temperature up to its new set level. The rise in the set point is due to the action of **pyrogens**, chemical agents that have the ability to readjust the hypothalamus. Pyrogens include various toxins, including proteins or their degraded products, and some endotoxins from bacteria, e.g. the **lipopolysaccharide** (LPS) layer from outside the cell wall of Gram-negative organisms. After death of the organism, the endotoxin is phagocytosed and the phagocyte itself (usually a macrophage) releases the chemical interleukin 1. This agent passes to the brain, where it appears to stimulate the formation of one of the prostaglandins, which in turn acts to reset the set point of the hypothalamus to a higher level. This is a rapid process, the temperature rising within 8–10 minutes of the release of interleukin 1. The endotoxin LPS only needs to cause the production of a few nanograms of interleukin 1 to cause fever. The involvement of prostaglandins is interesting, since this may explain how antipyretics such as aspirin and paracetamol may help to reduce the body temperature. These drugs block prostaglandin production (from a cell wall component called arachidonic acid), and may therefore prevent the effects of interleukin 1 on the hypothalamus.

Hyperthermia is a group of high body temperature disorders that includes **heat stroke** (Edwards 1998; Harker and Gibson 1995). This is a rapid rise in body temperature (to 40°C or more) caused by exposure to a hot environment in which the body temperature rises quickly, the hypothalamic set point is soon exceeded, but sweating fails to control the temperature and the casualty collapses. Symptoms include hot, dry skin, full and bounding pulse, headaches, confusion, dizziness and failing consciousness. The **penguin effect** is a similar heat stroke syndrome caused by a reduced ability to sweat in the centre of a tightly packed crowd. Examples of this occur in crowds at a major event, like a pop music concert, or people packed together in a commuter train on a hot day. It is named after penguins, which crowd together to conserve heat in Antarctica. Emotional excitement, dancing and, possibly, drugs are features at pop concerts that cause excess heat production with reduced ability to sweat. On crowded commuter transport, standing passengers may collapse but remain pinned upright, risking a loss of life. The penguin effect can cause many casualties at once, all suffering from the heat and also from fluid and electrolyte imbalance (Blows 1998). **Heat exhaustion** is associated with exposure to hot environments where the hypothalamus has been able to keep the temperature at relatively normal levels for most of the time by sweating. However, continued heat exposure and profuse sweating result in excessive fluid and electrolyte losses, which eventually leads to collapse with headaches, weak and rapid pulse, confusion, nausea, cramps and pallor. **Malignant hyperthermia** is a complication associated with an inherited muscular disorder triggered by administration of inhalant anaesthetics and muscle-relaxing drugs, mostly in the young. The muscles maintain a state of contraction soon after induction of anaesthesia, and this muscle activity generates heat which can raise the body temperature by as much as 1°C every 5 minutes. About 20% of sufferers can die from the effects as it also induces acidosis, tachycardia and hypotension.

Febrile convulsions in children under 7 years of age indicate two things: a pyrexia usually caused by an infection and a hypothalamus that is too immature to cope with the high temperature. The most common causes are chest and ear infections, both of which will require investigation, but any infection can trigger a fit at this age. The mechanism that responds to a high temperature by causing a fit is poorly understood. Clearly, however, the management is two pronged: treating and terminating the fit quickly, which involves reducing the temperature, followed by investigating and treating the underlying infection. Preventative measures carried out by the parents at home or nurses in hospital are beneficial and require early detection of pyrexia and cooling the child gently before a fit is triggered. Here, thermometers are not so important. Most homes do not have them, and many parents probably do not know how to use them properly. It is usually sufficient for worried parents to feel the child's head and trunk and recognise that the child has a high temperature. It then becomes more important to remove excess clothing, cool down the environment if it is too hot and get medical help rather than worry about measuring the child's temperature. In the clinical environment accurate measurement becomes important and is easily achieved. In all cases of febrile convulsion, reassuring the parents is as much part of the treatment as is managing the fit, and includes allowing the parents access to the child at the earliest opportunity and for as long as possible to allay any fears raised about epilepsy, which is only a very rare complication.

In any of the cases of excessive heat disorder, treatment has traditionally involved cooling along with fluid and electrolyte replacement where necessary. Reducing the high temperature is problematic since cooling too rapidly can induce shock and shivering, which would cause more heat production. It has been generally accepted for years that the temperature should be reduced gradually, i.e. at a rate no faster than 1°C per hour, although in practice this has often been difficult to achieve and record. Tepid sponging is most often adopted on the understanding that adding water to the skin promotes heat loss by evaporation. Recent evidence on this, however, is that sponging to reduce fever, especially in children, is probably counterproductive since it causes the body to generate heat through shivering and is uncomfortable for the child (Blumenthal 1998; Anon. 1999). Given that fever is a normal body response to infection or inflammation, there is a growing volume of literature indicating that aggressive (or rapid) efforts to reduce the temperature may not be beneficial and could cause unwanted difficulties (Edwards 1998; Harker and Gibson 1995). This creates a vacuum in terms of what to do for a febrile child or adult. This question becomes critical to parents faced with a febrile child at 2 a.m. Biologically, there are some basic principles that may help us. In general, provided they are sweating, adults cope with high temperatures better than children because of the maturity of the hypothalamus. Sweating is a sign that the hypothalamus is still doing its job. Children below 7 years of age are the most likely to suffer convulsions, so it may be prudent to try and prevent the temperature from going very high in this age group. Removal of all unnecessary clothing and providing a cool environment to promote natural heat loss is a useful approach. Cool drinks are of value because they reach the core temperature quickly and replace lost fluids. For this, however, it is vital that the child is conscious and able to swallow. Be aware of the risk of shivering and try to prevent this since shivering is an indication that the body has lost heat too quickly and is trying to generate more heat to combat the loss. A controlled environmental temperature is critical. Electric fans help to cool the environment if this is hot but should never be aimed directly at the sufferer since this would cool the periphery and send impulses of cold sensation from thermal receptors in the skin to the brain. These impulses may be misleading to the hypothalamus, which then tries to prevent heat loss from the body and generate more heat. Also, cold air from a fan could cause peripheral vasoconstriction, which then prevents heat transfer by blood from the core to the skin. Although tepid sponging is not generally recommended, it is probably a valid technique when applied to the hyperpyrexic patient who has lost the ability to sweat, i.e. the patient is hot and dry. Failure to sweat suggests that the hypothalamus has failed to respond, probably because the set point has been adjusted to a much higher level than normal. Antipyretic drugs, e.g. paracetamol, have a role to play in the management of elevated temperatures in persons who are capable of taking oral medication, especially children. They block the formation of prostaglandins, which promote elevation of the temperature, as noted earlier (p. 18). Aspirin is a useful antipyretic, but it should never be given to children below the age of 12 years as this can induce Reye's syndrome, a severe neurological disorder that is known to follow viral illnesses, such as influenza, colds or chicken pox, which have been treated with this drug. Antipyretics alone are unlikely to prevent febrile convulsions, and other measures are required.

Abnormal cold body temperatures

Exposure to cold leads to a general loss of body heat, known as **hypothermia**, or a local heat loss, called **frostbite**. Hypothermia can happen in anyone, but the largest numbers of cases occur in the extremes of age: the very young and the very old. This is due again to problems with the hypothalamus. In the very young it is still immature and cannot fully control temperature balance. Below the age at which they crawl, babies can lose heat rapidly without the benefit of the major muscles generating heat by activity. Lying or sitting, without the ability to move or change position, does not allow much production of muscle heat energy. Babies compensate for this with **brown fat** that can generate heat, particularly when stimulated by melatonin, a hormone produced from serotonin in the pineal gland of the brain. Brown fat is largely lost with increasing age as the child becomes a lot more physically active. Very young children may not have developed the ability to shiver, and they cannot therefore gain heat from this mechanism. Despite the warming effect of brown fat, children exposed to prolonged or excessive cold will suffer from hypothermia. They feel cold to the touch and they may shiver, especially older children. They may also appear limp and quiet, and may have cyanosed lips and extremities. They can collapse and possibly die from respiratory or cardiac failure if they are not protected against both the external cold and their own heat loss. Wet children are especially vulnerable after swimming or playing in water. Because of poor insulation caused by very little body hair, the human baby is very vulnerable and is dependent on warm environments and the insulation provided by clothing. **Incubators** have saved the lives of many newborn babies who are unable to sustain normothermia by their own volition, e.g. such babies as **preterm** or **failure to thrive**.

Incubation maintains the infants environmental temperature usually a few degrees higher than average body temperature until it is mature enough to stabilise its own homeostatic control of heat loss. Since incubators must be opened occasionally to allow essential access, the room temperature must also be warm enough to prevent sudden chilling of the infant.

The elderly undergo age-related changes to many body systems, including the brain, and the hypothalamus gradually declines in function as neurones are lost. The temperature control centre becomes less able to respond to body temperature changes quickly and cannot always provide comprehensive heat regulation when environmental temperatures are above or below average for prolonged periods of time. Although hot environments can be harmful to the elderly, who can die in a heat wave, it is the cold that causes the most problems and the most deaths. Cold weather kills many elderly people annually, and special consideration must be given to older people during winter months who live alone in poorly heated homes. It is worse for those with limited mobility and those who are vulnerable to falling. An old person lying injured on a floor will lose heat quickly from his/her large surface area and may die from hypothermia before being found. Of the two age groups, it is probably true to say that children will suffer from the effects of cold quickly, whereas elderly people gradually deteriorate as a result of prolonged cold exposure.

An important cause of hypothermia is surgery: during the **perioperative period** patients are exposed to cool environments and suffer a significant body temperature loss. Intensive care may also put some patients at risk of hypothermia, mainly because patients are inactive (thus not generating much heat), they may be exposed for medical and nursing procedures and their total energy input for the day may be considerably less than what their body is used to. In these specialised clinical areas many units carry out **total temperature management (TTM)**, as a means of preventing hypothermia. This involves continual monitoring of the patient's core temperature by electronic probes placed inside the body, in sites such as the pulmonary artery, oesophagus, rectum or urinary bladder. The temperature can be read at any time as a digital figure on a screen that shows other physiological readings. TTM also involves maintenance of normothermia in the patient during lengthy exposure or surgery using specialised electrically warmed blankets. It also involves very strict control of the environmental temperature, often at a higher than average level, and rewarming of fluids or blood before, or during, intravenous infusion, again with specialised equipment designed with fluid-rewarming systems.

Clearly the hypothermia sufferer needs to be warmer, but the problems associated with the treatment of hypothermia are about the process of rewarming. The danger lies with the low core temperature at which the vital organs must try to function. Any attempt to rewarm the person by applying heat to the periphery, i.e. warming up the skin, can be counterproductive and dangerous. The use of heat close to the skin, e.g. hot water bottles or the close proximity of heaters, will make the person look better and feel warmer to touch, but they only serve to dilate peripheral blood vessels, which then take vital blood, and therefore heat, away from the core, cooling the core temperature further. This is not the same as using the specialised heated blankets identified in TTM, when the core temperature is essentially normal, and the emphasis is on preventing hypothermia, not treating it. The main points about rewarming the established hypothermia are that the person involved must first be urgently removed to a warmer environment to prevent further heat loss. Trying to rewarm someone in a very cold environment is an uphill struggle that the patient may lose. In addition, any wet clothing must be removed and the skin dried. Water on the skin acts like sweating in removing further heat quickly. The body should then be covered in dry clothing and the person preferably put to bed. Warm drinks with sugar given to the conscious person who is still able to swallow would be beneficial. Monitoring of the temperature by an electronic thermometer or low-scale mercury thermometer may be better achieved via a route other than oral or axilla routes. The oral route may be dangerous in a patient who is in an altered state of consciousness, and axillary routes will only give peripheral temperature results. Rewarming, like cooling of pyrexia, should be gradual: often quoted as 1°C rise per hour. Rapid rewarming, like rapid cooling, is harmful as it can induce shock. It is not possible to raise the core temperature quickly, and any attempts to do so, like using warm or hot baths, will only warm the peripheral temperature causing dilation of the skin vessels, which in turn causes cardiovascular collapse. Once cooled, the core temperature is only warmed by heat produced from tissue metabolism, and this will take time to be effective.

Thermal injury

Frostbite is a local thermal injury, and as such it is akin to burns because tissue is destroyed by an extreme temperature abnormality. The intense local cold causes vasoconstriction to the point of occlusion of blood flow, with resultant anoxia of dependent tissues. All cellular metabolism stops when oxygen and nutrient delivery is shut down, wastes accumulate in the cells and enzymic reactions can no longer function. Apart from cold, early signs of frostbite can include paraesthesia (tingling sensations) and numbness, and pallor of the affected tissues, which may turn blue (cyanosis) and ultimately black. This is when the tissues are dead (**necrosis** or gangrene) and may slough off. An infection of the area involved can then follow with life-threatening results. If the tissues involved survive and recover, they become red, blistered and painful. Emergency treatment involves prevention of the condition worsening by removable to a warmer environment as soon as possible and gentle rewarming by placing the affected parts against warmer areas of the body. Removal of any tight clothing or restrictive jewellery is essential to promote good blood flow and to avoid rubbing the injury, which can cause tissue trauma. Light dressings may help, and medical treatment is usually essential. Frostbite will mostly affect toes and fingers because these parts are at the distal extremes of the cardiovascular system, i.e. they are at the point of lowest tissue perfusion pressure (the mean arterial pressure, or MAP, see p. 54) and therefore will suffer more damaging vasoconstriction for less environmental temperature drop than those parts closer to the heart. Also, distal extremities are thinner than central parts (compare the thickness of a toe with that of the thigh or the trunk) and therefore cold can penetrate extremities faster, i.e. they have less body mass per unit of surface area than thicker parts of the body. Since it is the surface area that is exposed to the cold, it has less mass of tissue below it to chill than the same surface area of, for example, the thigh. This smaller mass of tissue is not capable of heat production to counteract the cold on the same scale as bulkier parts. The distal extremities are more dependent on heat delivered by the blood than any other parts of the body. This is why feet can get cold quickly and hot water bottles are used by some people to warm their feet in bed. It is also the reason why the temperature of extremities is a good indication of the status of the circulation in that limb. The warm hand or foot has a good circulation, whereas cold extremities indicate poor circulation. This is a useful observation on limbs encased in plaster casts or where an injury or vascular complication may disturb blood flow to that extremity. Using hand or foot temperature to assess the circulation on the unaffected side will identify what the normal circulatory state is at that time, and given both limbs are normally equal this will indicate what the circulatory state should be in the affected limb. Such a comparison made between the good limb and the affected limb may identify a serious problem that requires urgent attention, e.g. possibly the plaster or bandages are too tight.

Key points

- Body temperature is generally stabilised at 37°C, with a homeostatic negative feedback mechanism in place to ensure this.
- The hypothalamus in the base of the brain is the central control of this mechanism, with input from temperature-sensitive sensory nerve endings in the skin and around vital organs.
- Normally the body gains heat by cellular metabolism from energy-rich food and loses heat by evaporation of sweat, elimination, conduction, convection and radiation.
- Sweating is the main mechanism of heat loss and is a cardinal sign of overheating (pyrexia).
- Shivering is the main mechanism of heat gain and is a cardinal sign of the body being too cold (hypothermia).
- The core temperature is the most accurate to record since this is the temperature at which the vital organs must function.
- The peripheral temperature is usually lower than the core temperature since it responds more to the ambient temperature and humidity.
- Mercury-in-glass thermometers are subject to hazards, from broken glass, mercury vapour and cross-infection, and are being replaced in most clinical areas.
- Disposable, electronic and infrared thermometers are gaining wider clinical use.
- Younger children are more vulnerable to temperature changes and may suffer febrile convulsions. The optimum method of temperature recording in small children is via the rectal route.
- Electric fans are useful for cooling the environment but must not be directed at the patient.
- Tepid sponging may be uncomfortable for the patient and may be of little value except in those circumstances of rapid body temperature rise where sweating has failed to control body temperature.

- Rewarming in hypothermia, like cooling in pyrexia, should be gradual, often quoted as 1°C rise per hour. Rapid rewarming, like rapid cooling, is harmful as it can induce shock.
- The temperature of extremities is a good indication of the status of the circulation in that limb. The warm hand or foot has a good circulation, whereas cold extremities indicate a poorer circulation.

References

Anon. (1996) Mercury or modern? *Community Nurse*, 2(10): 25–26.

Anon. (1999) Fever analysis remains a burning issue. *Nursing Times*, 95(9): 47.

Blows W. T. (1998) Crowd Physiology: the 'penguin effect'. *Accident and Emergency Nursing*, 6: 126–129.

Blumenthal I. (1998) What parents think of fever. *Family Practice*, 15(6): 513–518.

Davis K. (1993) The accuracy of typanic temperature measurement in children. *Pediatric Nursing*, 19(3): 267–272.

Edwards S. L. (1998) High Temperature. *Professional Nurse*, 13(8): 521–526.

Erickson R. S., Meyer L. T. and Woo T. M. (1996) Accuracy of chemical dot thermometers in critically ill adults and young children. *Image: Journal of Nursing Scholarship*, 28(1): 23–28.

Guyton A. and Hall J. (1996) *Textbook of Medical Physiology*. W. B. Saunders, Philadelphia.

Harker J. and Gibson P. (1995) Heat-stroke: a review of rapid cooling techniques. *Intensive and Critical Care Nursing*, 11: 198–202.

Henker R., Kramer D. and Rogers S. (1997) Fever. *AACN Clinical Issues*, 8(3): 351–367.

Morley C. (1992) Why taking temperatures rectally is right. *Paediatric Nursing*, 4(6): 7.

Morley C. J., Hewson P. H., Thornton A. J. and Cole T. J. (1992) Axillary and rectal temperature measurements in infants. *Archives of Disease in Childhood*, 67: 122–125.

O'Toole S. (1998) Temperature measuring devices. *Professional Nurse*, 13(11): 779–786.

Watson R. (1998) Controlling body temperature in adults. *Nursing Standard*, 12(20): 49–55.

Chapter 2

Cardiovascular observations (I): the pulse

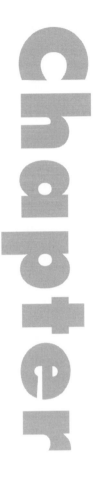

- Introduction
- Blood physiology
- Heart physiology
- Observations of the pulse, apex beat, electrocardiogram and heart sounds
- The effects of cardiovascular drugs
- The pulse in children
- Key points

Introduction

The need to move many substances from one part of the body to another is vital to the very existence of the individual. The blood has the task of transporting:

1 water and nutrients from the digestive system to the cells;
2 oxygen from the lungs to the cells;
3 carbon dioxide from the cells to the lungs;
4 wastes from the cells to the kidneys;
5 defensive cells from the bone marrow to sites of infection;
6 hormones from the glands to the cells;
7 antibodies from lymphocytes to antigens;
8 proteins from the liver to all parts of the circulatory system, and much more.

Moving a liquid like blood requires a pump; and so we have a heart. The heart cycle creates two parameters that we can measure: the number of times it beats per minute, recorded as a pulse, and the pressure of blood leaving the heart, known simply as blood pressure. These are inseparably linked; the pulse is dependent on blood pressure since it is the pressure of blood exerted against the arterial wall in waves. Similarly, the pulse varies with the blood pressure, i.e. if the blood pressure falls the pulse rate rises to compensate, since too low a pressure will deliver inadequate blood to the tissues, and the heart will try to speed up the delivery. Measuring these two parameters alone will give great insight into the system that delivers life to the tissues and therefore provides an understanding of the basic state of the body.

Blood physiology

Blood is a liquid tissue, having a water-based extracellular component (the plasma) housing cells which themselves contain water. The cells are red (**red blood cells** or **RBCs**, also called **erythrocytes**), white (**white blood cells** or **WBCs**, also called **leucocytes**) and small cell fragments called **platelets** (or **thrombocytes**) (Figure 2.1). Red cells carry **haemoglobin**, which binds the respiratory gases oxygen and carbon dioxide (see Chapter 3). Like all blood cells, erythrocytes are developed in **bone marrow**, but as mature cells they have no nucleus and therefore their survival in circulation is only about 120 days. They are continually being replaced by new ones from the bone marrow. White cells last longer, and their role is to fight infection: part of the

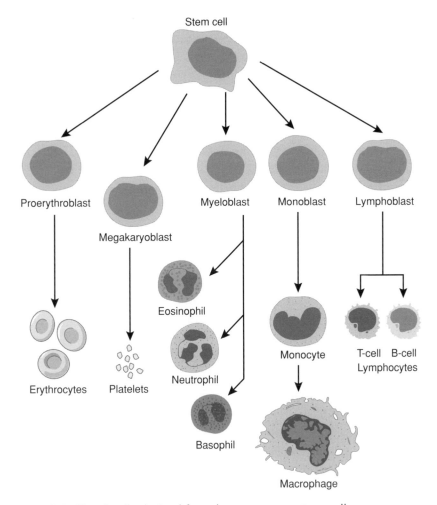

FIGURE 2.1 Blood cells derived from bone marrow stem cells.

body's defence strategy. Several kinds of WBCs exist: **lymphocytes**, which use various mechanisms to kill invading organisms (**antigens**); **monocytes**, which are **phagocytic**, i.e. they engulf and destroy antigens; and various **granulocytes**, which release important chemicals as part of the defensive role. Platelets help to control blood loss when injury to blood vessels occurs, either by blocking minute holes in the vessel wall if the injury is microscopic or by triggering the blood-clotting mechanism.

Red cells have a combination of two **antigens** (i.e. proteins capable of provoking an immune reaction) on their surface: **antigens A** and **B**. If the red cells have only antigen A, this is **blood group A**; cells with only antigen B produce **blood group B**; antigens A and B together create **blood group AB**, and no antigen is **blood group O. Antibodies** are present in the plasma (immune proteins that react with antigens), but clearly individuals cannot have the antibodies that react with their own antigen; instead, they have antibodies that react with *other* antigens (see Table 2.1).

A second type of RBC surface antigen, the D-factor, gives rise to the **rhesus factor**. If the D-factor is present, the blood is **rhesus (Rh) positive**, and the plasma has no **anti-D antibody**. If the D-factor is absent, the blood is **rhesus (Rh) negative**, and the plasma has **anti-D antibody**. Any of the four ABO groups can be either Rh positive or Rh negative, i.e. eight blood groups in all. In all these cases the plasma antigens cannot react with their own red cells, but **transfusion** of blood from one person to another creates the conditions which could cause a reaction, and this must be avoided. **Haemolysis** is one type of reaction where red cells are destroyed, **haemoglobin** is released and the patient can suffer severe **anaemia** with **jaundice**. **Agglutination** is another type of reaction where red cells clump together in large lumps which can block smaller vessels, such as the arterioles within the kidneys, causing kidney failure. These are **mismatched** transfusions, and careful checking is required to prevent this (Figure 2.2).

Of the eight transported substances listed in the introduction, oxygen and carbon dioxide are mostly carried by the haemoglobin of the RBCs; the WBCs are the defensive cells. All the remaining substances are carried in the plasma: some dissolved and some in suspension. The end products of digestion and inhaled oxygen are transported to the tissues, the waste products and carbon dioxide are carried to the excretory organs and whole proteins, called **plasma proteins**, remain in the blood. Plasma proteins have many functions, for example as **antibodies** (produced by lymphocytes and known as **immunoglobulins**, or Ig), which help to fight infections; albumin, which aids the return of tissue fluid to the plasma; and clotting factors, which are essential for blood clot formation. The blood also distributes heat to all parts of the body, especially from the core to the periphery (see Chapter 1).

TABLE 2.1 Blood groups and antigens

Blood group	Antigen on RBC	Antibodies in plasma
A	A	Anti-B (reacts with B antigen)
B	B	Anti-A (reacts with A antigen)
AB	A + B	No antibodies
O	No antigens	Anti-A + anti-B (reacts with both)

Recipient blood

Donor blood		A Anti-B antibody	B Anti-A antibody	AB None	O Anti-A + anti-B antibodies
	A	✓	✗	✓	✗
	B	✗	✓	✓	✗
	AB	✗	✗	✓	✗
	O	✓	✓	✓	✓

Figure 2.2 The ABO blood groups compatibility grid. The donor's red cells (A and B antigens) are matched with the recipient's plasma (anti-A and anti-B antibodies) to identify any dangerous reaction (×) or no reaction (✓). Recipient AB can take blood from any group (universal recipient) and donor O can give blood to any group (universal donor) provided the rhesus factor (not shown) is compatible.

Heart physiology

The heart is a muscular pump divided vertically by a wall, the **septum**, into separate left and right sides (Figure 2.3) (Vickers 1999a). Each side has a smaller upper chamber, the **atrium** (plural **atria**), and a larger lower chamber, the **ventricle**. Valves exist in a line between the atria and ventricles, the **atrioventricular (AV)** valves, which close to prevent backflow of blood during heart contraction. These are the **bicuspid** (bi = two, cuspid = cusps or flaps) valve on the left and the **tricuspid** (tri = three) valve on the right. Blood is received into the right atrium from the **vena cavae**, the major veins returning blood from the body to the right side of the heart. On the left side, the atrium receives blood from the **pulmonary veins** returning blood from the lungs. From both the atria blood passes through the AV valves and fills the ventricles. Contraction of these ventricles pushes blood through **semilunar valves,** which prevent backflow to the ventricles: the **aortic valve** on the left and **pulmonary valve** on the right. The **aorta** is the main artery taking blood from the left side of the heart for distribution around the body.

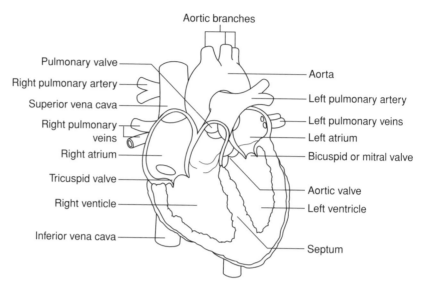

Aortic branches

Pulmonary valve

Right pulmonary artery

Superior vena cava

Right pulmonary veins

Right atrium

Tricuspid valve

Right venticle

Inferior vena cava

Aorta

Left pulmonary artery

Left pulmonary veins

Left atrium

Bicuspid or mitral valve

Aortic valve

Left ventricle

Septum

FIGURE 2.3 Cross-section through the heart (viewed anteriorly).

The first branches of the aorta are the **coronary arteries**, which supply the heart wall itself with blood. Partial or complete blockage of these arteries deprives the myocardium of blood, leading to angina or myocardial infarction (both forms of heart attack, see p. 62). The **pulmonary artery** carries blood from the right side of the heart to the lungs for oxygenation. The result is a double circulation, i.e. a **systemic** circulation from the left side of the heart to the tissues and back to the right heart, and a **pulmonary** circulation from the right side of the heart to the lungs and back to the left heart (Figure 2.4). The systemic circulation is much larger, involving all the systems of the body, and is sustained at a high pressure of blood. The much smaller pulmonary system operates at lower pressures because blood has only to pass from the heart to the lungs and back; entirely within the chest.

The heart wall consists of a muscle layer, the **myocardium**, an inner smooth lining of **epithelium**, the **endocardium**, and an outer membrane, the **pericardium**. The myocardium has specialised cells that are linked by branches, and this allows them to contract simultaneously, acting as a single unit, or **functional syncytium**. Myocardial cells contract during stimulation by nerve impulses that pass through the heart from the **sinoatrial (SA) node**, the pacemaker of the heart, which can trigger regular cardiac contractions without outside control (an *inherent power of rhythmic contraction*). The SA node has external regulation by the **autonomic nervous system (ANS)**,

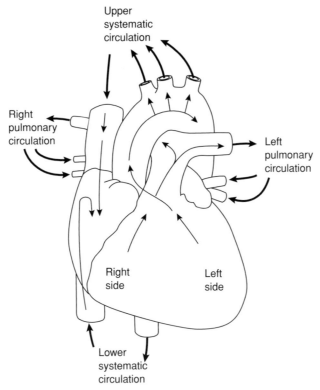

Upper systematic circulation

Right pulmonary circulation

Left pulmonary circulation

Right side

Left side

Lower systematic circulation

FIGURE 2.4 Double circulation of the blood from the heart. The systemic circulation passes from the aorta to the upper and lower parts of the body. The pulmonary circulation passes from the pulmonary arteries to the left and right lungs.

which maintains the heart rate at an average level (about 72 beats per minute). The **sympathetic** component of the ANS increases the heart rate, whereas the **parasympathetic** component (via the **vagus nerve**) decreases the heart rate (Vickers 1999b). They work together to stabilise the heart rate, but at the same time the presence of both sympathetic and parasympathetic components allows the heart rate to be increased or decreased as the tissues demand for blood changes. During activity, limb muscles in particular force an increase in heart rate to supply more blood, and the sympathetic component will be dominant. At rest, especially during sleep, the parasympathetic component dominates to slow the heart rate down.

The **cardiac cycle** (Vickers 1999c) is the sequence of events the heart goes through from one beat to the next. Contraction of the ventricles is a **systole**, when blood is pushed out of the heart, followed by ventricular relaxation, or **diastole**, the refilling phase. These events are linked to the electrical conduction activity that starts at the SA node and passes through the myocardium. As it crosses the **atria** they contract and push some blood downwards to top up the ventricles. The impulse arrives at the level of the AV valves, but it does not progress beyond this. At this level the next node, the **AV node**, comes in to play. This node picks up the impulse and transmits it down the ventricular septum via conduction tissue called the **bundle of His**, which divides into the left and right **bundle branches**. From the lower end of the septum, the impulse passes via the **Purkinje fibres** at the end of the bundle branches to the ventricular muscle. The impulse passes upwards across the ventricles causing them to contract (Figure 2.5). Regulation of the heart is maintained by the **cardiac centre**, one of the *vital centres* in a part of the brain called the **medulla** within the **brain stem**. If any injury or disorder were to affect the cardiac centre the heart would stop beating immediately.

The **cardiac output (CO)** is the **heart rate (HR)** multiplied by the **stroke volume (SV)**, i.e. CO = HR × SV. This formula is the volume of blood pumped out of a single ventricle in 1 minute. Each time a ventricle contracts about 70 ml of blood is pushed into the arteries (the stroke volume). The ventricles contract on average 72 times per minute (the heart rate); so the cardiac output per ventricle is 70 ml multiplied by 72 beats per minute, i.e. 5,040 ml per minute. The cardiac output per ventricle is just over 5,000 ml. Considering the total blood volume in circulation is on average about 5,000 ml, it means that each ventricle pushes out the entire blood volume every minute.

Observations of the pulse, apex beat, electrocardiogram and heart sounds

The pulse rate and strength

The **pulse** is caused by pressure exerted on the arterial wall causing expansion of the vessel for the brief moment that the wave of pressure passes. The pressure wave is caused by contraction of the ventricles on the left side of the heart forcing blood into the arteries. The heart beats about 72 times per minute at rest, and so this becomes the average adult pulse rate. *All* arteries demonstrate a pulse, but they are not all accessible for observation. For clinical purposes, the **radial** pulse is mostly used. This is found on the inner aspect of the wrist, on the thumb (= radial) side of a ridge (a tendon) that runs almost centrally

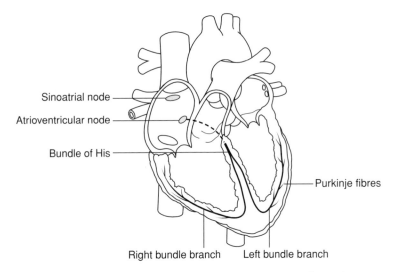

Figure 2.5 The cardiac conduction system. Impulses arise from the sinoatrial node and pass across the atria to the atrioventricular node. From here impulses pass down from the bundle of His (also called the atrioventricular bundle) and into the left bundle branch and right bundle branch. The Purkinje fibres are wide terminal branch cells that distribute the impulses to the myocardial cells.

down the distal end of the arm into the wrist. Pulses are normally taken by the observer's middle three fingers, not the thumb. Taking the radial pulse is acceptable because it is non-invasive, not embarrassing and for the most part accurate. It only loses accuracy when the blood pressure drops too low, or the arm is too obese to allow palpation of the pulse. Other pulse sites are possible, but they are associated with difficulties and are reserved for specific circumstances (Figure 2.6). The **brachial** pulse occurs along the inner aspect of the upper arm, beneath the brachial muscle, feeling the pulse against the **humerus** (upper arm bone). The **temporal** pulse can be found on each side of the head just anterior to the upper margin of the ear. The **femoral** pulse is about midway across the groin and is used sometimes as a pulse check during cardiac arrest procedures, when embarrassment of the patient is not an issue. The **carotid** pulse lies in the soft tissues on each side of the larynx and is also used in cardiac arrest. Using this pulse on conscious patients, as may sometimes be necessary if the radial pulse is obscure, requires an explanation so that the patient will not be concerned. This pulse must be felt with only gentle pressure, since the carotid artery is part of the blood supply to the brain and must not be obstructed. The **pedal** (= foot) pulses, mainly the **posterior tibial** and the **dorsalis pedis**

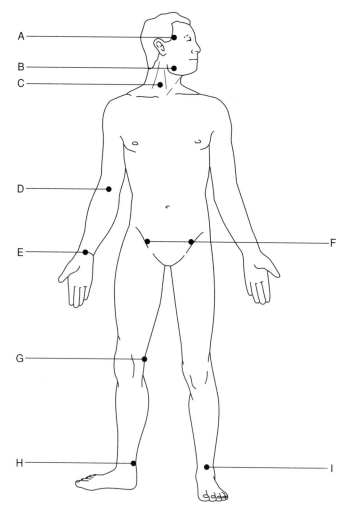

FIGURE 2.6 Arterial pulse sites on the body. A, temporal; B, facial (on jaw); C, common carotid; D, brachial; E, radial (thumb side, the usual pulse for clinical practice); F, right and left femoral; G, popliteal (behind the knee); H, posterior tibial; I, dorsalis pedis (see Figure 2.7 for H and I).

(Figure 2.7), are important for assessing the blood supply to the leg and foot and should be used in any limb vascular disease or during the management of all lower limb injuries and during surgery. They are also essential after any application of potentially restrictive treatments, such as support bandages or splintage material, especially if limb swelling is still likely.

The pulse rate is normally elevated during exercise and hard physical labour, and a fast rate is also part of the response to fear and excitement. **Tachycardia** is a fast pulse rate, e.g. 100 beats per minute or more, and

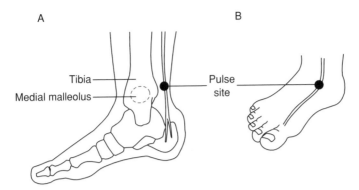

FIGURE 2.7 Pedal (foot) pulses. A, post-tibial artery (immediately behind the medial malleolus on the tibia); B, dorsalis pedis (on the top of the foot midway between the lateral and medial malleolli).

bradycardia is a slow rate, usually below 50 beats per minute. The normal maximum heart rate is about 180 beats per minute, i.e. the maximum above which normal filling of the heart cannot take place. At this rate the entire cardiac cycle lasts just 0.33 seconds. The difference in the systolic and diastolic phases at heart rates of 67 and 180 beats per minute (bpm) are:

	Heart rate 67 bpm	Heart rate 180 bpm
Systole	0.35 seconds	0.2 seconds
Diastole	0.58 seconds	0.13 seconds

To achieve adequate ventricular filling during diastole requires a minimum diastolic phase of about 0.12 seconds, so heart rates above 180 beats per minute would reduce the diastolic phase below this minimum, and the cardiac output would be reduced.

Tachycardia is a feature of systemic infections, especially associated with fever, and is a compensatory mechanism for improving the tissue blood supply when a patient is in shock. Bradycardia can occur during **heart block**, i.e. when the impulse from the SA node does not always reach the ventricles, and the ventricular contraction rate slows down.

The strength of the pulse is dependent on two factors: the force applied to the blood by the left ventricle during contraction and the stroke volume. The force of contraction can vary normally and in diseases such as **left heart failure (LVF)**, where the myocardium is unable to achieve a full stroke volume (Gordon and Child 2000a,b). Excess blood may be retained inside the heart at the end of each systolic phase. This can result in a reduced output to the arteries (the **forward**

problem) and a backlog of blood unable to enter the ventricles because they are partly filled already and can only accept a limited blood volume from the veins (the **backward problem**) (see p. 81). The stroke volume will decline in **hypovolaemic shock** (hypo = below normal, vol = volume, aemic = blood), where the blood volume in circulation is less than normal as a result of bleeding or burns. A weak, rapid pulse is characteristic of shock: weak due to a low stroke volume, and rapid because the heart tries to compensate by pumping faster, which is part of the sympathetic response. **Thyrotoxicosis** (raised blood levels of thyroxin) and heart block can increase the force of contraction. **Palpitations** are heart beats felt by the patient on the chest wall. They may be associated with arrhythmias but are often normal, being caused by extreme exercise or occasional extra beats.

Apex beat

The radial pulse rate taken at the wrist is a record of the number of times the left ventricle contracts per minute. So another way to measure this would be to listen through the chest wall, via a stethoscope, to the heart itself, counting the sounds per minute. It is important to listen to the ventricle (usually the left) at the outermost and lowest point of the heart (the apex of the heart); this is known as the **apex beat**. The radial pulse and heart sounds should be equal in number, but sometimes the ventricular contraction is so weak that the force is insufficient to create a pulse at the wrist. The difference between the radial and apex beats can be measured by two nurses working together. One takes the radial pulse in the usual way while the other listens to the apex beat. This is found by placing the diaphragm of a stethoscope over the space between the left fifth and sixth ribs close to the **midclavicular line**, an imaginary line drawn down the chest from a point midway along the left clavicle. Using the same watch and counting over the same 60 seconds, both the radial and the apex beats are recorded. Any deficit may show an apex beat higher than the radial beat, and subtracting the later from the former the deficit can be calculated. In an example of an apex beat of 84 and a radial pulse of 74 the difference is 10 beats, i.e. the ventricles have had ten contractions during that minute that were not strong enough to create a radial pulse. Sometimes the radial count is recorded as higher than the apex beat, but this is not possible since the radial pulse depends on ventricular contractions. This result is clearly an error and the observation should be repeated.

The electrocardiogram (ECG)

Willem Einthoven (1860–1927), a Dutch physiologist, was awarded the 1924 Nobel prize for physiology for pioneering **electro-cardiography**. In 1909 Augustus Waller demonstrated to the Royal Society in London the recording of an **electrocardiogram (ECG)** from a pet dog called Jimmie (Levick 1992). This procedure is an important fast, accurate, non-invasive means of diagnosis of cardiac disease that can be carried out almost anywhere. The ECG records the electrical activity of the heart muscle as it occurs at skin level having passed through the extracellular fluid between the heart and the body surface. Electrical activity (called **depolarisation**) at the SA and AV nodes is too small to create recordable changes at the skin surface, but the electrical activity within the larger myocardial muscle bulk can be recorded throughout repeated heart cycles. The tracing represents different views of the heart, like seeing different aspects of the same object when viewed from varying angles. The leads attached to the patient provide these different views of the heart (Figure 2.8). The recording is a measure of the electrical difference between one electrode and another (i.e. bipolar = two leads used) in leads I, II, III, aVR, aVL

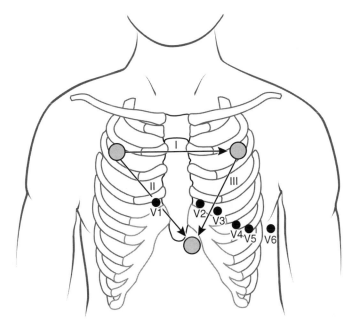

FIGURE 2.8 ECG lead positions I, II, III and V1 to V6.

and aVF (see Figure 2.8). The V leads use a free-moving electrode placed at specific sites on the chest wall that measure the electrical activity at each site (i.e. unipolar = one roving lead). The main direction of electrical flow through the heart, called the **electrical axis**, runs down the heart from the SA node to the ventricles. This varies between individuals in positions between the direction of leads I and aVF. The chest leads, therefore, are snapshots of this axis seen differently from these various views. The baseline of the tracing is **isoelectric**, i.e. zero voltage. Any deflection above this line indicates a view looking in the direction of the axis, i.e. positive (+), and a deflection below the baseline indicates a view that is more than 90° away from the axis, i.e. negative (–). The normal pattern of activity is known and abnormalities of the tracing can be detected and identified as specific heart disorders (Figure 2.9). Atrial depolarisation (normally accompanied by atrial contraction) is recorded on the ECG as the P wave, followed by the PQ interval, an isoelectric event as the impulse passes down the bundle of His. The QRS complex is the depolarisation event of the ventricles (ventricular contraction, or systole), followed by ventricular repolarisation, the T wave (ventricular relaxation) (Vickers 1999b). **Sinus rhythm** is the term given to a normal ECG pattern. **Arrhythmias** are deviations of the ECG pattern seen in various cardiac disorders and are used to aid the diagnosis, e.g. **ectopic beats,** which are extra systoles generated within the damaged ventricular myocardium after a myocardial infarction (Figure 2.9) (Hatchett *et al.* 1999).

Heart sounds

Auscultation (listening through a **stethoscope**) has traditionally been part of the doctor's examination of the patient, but now specialist cardiac nurses may train to observe for normal and abnormal heart sounds, and their identification is important.

The closure (*not* opening) of the heart valves causes normal heart sounds as the valve cusps vibrate. Several heart sounds are recognised: the first (said to sound like 'lubb...') is the closure of the AV valves (tri- and bicuspid valves), and the second (said to sound like 'dubb...') is the closure of the semilunar valves (aortic and pulmonary). If the aortic valve closes just before the pulmonary valve the second sound can be split into two sounds, as is common in healthy young people during inspiration. Breathing in causes increased filling of the right ventricle and therefore a raised right ventricular stroke volume. This

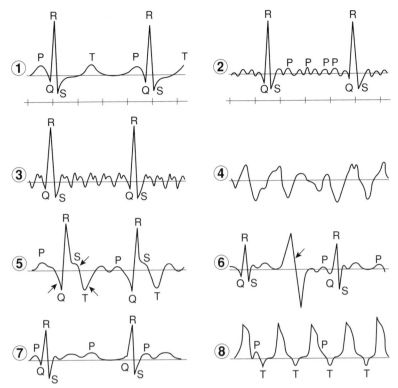

FIGURE 2.9 Normal and abnormal ECG tracings. 1, Normal sinus rhythm; 2, atrial fibrillation with multiple P waves between the QRS complexes; 3, atrial flutter with the saw tooth appearance between the QRS complex; 4, ventricular fibrillation, causes no cardiac output and requires urgent resuscitation; 5, myocardial infarction with large Q waves, ST elevation and inverted T waves; 6, ventricular extrasystole (ectopic beat); 7, heart block with P waves occurring at any point; 8, ventricular tachycardia with closer packed QRS complexes.

takes longer to eject during systole and the pulmonary valve closure is delayed. A third sound caused by the entry of blood into the relaxed ventricles at the start of diastole is also common in young people; a fourth sound is audible just before the first and is due to the atrial systole.

Valvular disorders create turbulence in the blood flow through the valve, and this disturbed flow causes extra sounds known as **murmurs**. **Stenosis** is a narrowing of the valve openings because the flaps will not part sufficiently to allow all the blood through. **Incompetence** occurs when a valve will not close properly and it allows backflow of blood, i.e. the valve is *leaky*. Since there are four valves and each is capable of either stenosis or incompetence, a total of eight disorders is possible, resulting in eight murmurs within the heart. But not all murmurs are due to disease. In young people, sometimes during pregnancy or in strenuous exercise, a **benign murmu**r can occasionally be heard due to turbulence of the blood leaving the heart, and this is not a problem.

The effects of cardiovascular drugs

Various cardiovascular drugs affect the pulse rate and the blood pressure, and knowledge of this is necessary when evaluating a patient's results. **Positive inotropic drugs** (e.g. the **cardiac glycosides**, especially **digoxin**, and the **phosphodiesterase inhibitors**, such as **milrinone**) increase the force of contraction and are therefore used in heart failure. Digoxin particularly causes slowing of the heart rate, and care must be taken not to allow the pulse rate to drop below 60 beats per minute. Bradycardia is a sign of **digoxin toxicity**, and nurses should check the patients pulse before administration of this drug. In addition, patients taking this drug, especially the elderly, should be observed for confusion, nausea and **coupled beats**, i.e. two pulse beats together followed by a pause.

   Beta-blocking drugs, such as **propranolol**, reduce the sympathetic stimulation of the heart and therefore slow the heart rate. These are used to treat angina, i.e. chest pain caused by restricted blood flow down the coronary arteries as a result of arterial disease.

   Antiarrhythmic drugs, e.g. **verapamil**, **procainamide** and **lignocaine**, suppress the incidence and intensity of cardiac arrhythmias, either **supraventricular** (= above the ventricles, i.e. the atria) or **ventricular**.

The pulse in children

The cardiovascular system in children must cope with its own growth while catering for increased demands on it as a result of growth in all other parts of the body. In children the heart rate range falls gradually from 110–160 beats per minute at less than 1 year of age to 60–100 at more than 12 years of age. Breathing causes more pronounced changes in the heart rate in children than in adults, a difference of up to 30 beats per minute, slowing down during inspiration and accelerating during expiration.

   It may be recommended in some paediatric units for the nurse to use the brachial or temporal pulse with the younger child, as this may be easier to find in a less than co-operative child, and will therefore be more accurate. For the older child, when co-operation by the child is achieved, the radial pulse can be used. Using the carotid pulse in children is not justified since it carries specific risks, as noted on p. 35, regarding the blood supply to the brain, and should not therefore be used in children of any age.

Rapid heart rates can be caused by heart failure, a complication of **congenital heart defects**. These are distortions of the heart anatomy which the child is born with. **Atrial** or **ventricular septal defects** (**ASDs** or **VSDs**, the so-called hole in the heart) abnormally allow blood to pass from one side of the heart to the other. If blood passes from the right ventricle to the left ventricle through a VSD, deoxygenated blood (i.e. it lacks oxygen) fails to go to the lungs for oxygenation from the right ventricle and is pumped by the left ventricle back to the body again. Efforts by the heart to improve the oxygen supply to the body result in an increase in the cardiac output, usually a rise in the heart rate. Ultimately, if this is not corrected, the heart can enlarge and fail.

Key points

- The total blood volume in circulation is 5,000 ml.
- The blood cells are erythrocytes (red blood cells), leucocytes (white blood cells) and thrombocytes (platelets).
- Blood group A has antigen A on the RBCs and anti-B antibodies in the plasma. Similarly, blood group B has antigen B with anti-A antibodies; blood group AB has antigens A and B and no antibodies, and blood group O has no antigen and anti-A and anti-B antibodies.
- The rhesus factor (D-factor) is present in rhesus (Rh) positive, the plasma has no anti-D antibody. The D-factor is absent in rhesus (Rh) negative, the plasma has anti-D antibody.
- The heart wall has a muscular myocardium, an inner endocardium, and an outer pericardium.
- The sinoatrial (SA) node can trigger cardiac contractions with external regulation by the sympathetic (increases the heart rate) and the parasympathetic nervous systems (vagus nerve, decreases the heart rate).
- The cardiac cycle consists of a systole (ventricular contraction) followed by diastole (ventricular relaxation)
- Electrical conduction starts at the SA node, passes through the atrial myocardium, which contracts; the AV node picks up the impulse and transmits it down the ventricular septum via the bundle of His,

and then the left and right bundle branches to the Purkinje fibres in the ventricular muscle, which then contracts.

- For clinical purposes the radial pulse is mostly used.
- The normal adult pulse rate is 65–72 beats per minute.
- Tachycardia is a fast pulse rate and bradycardia is a slow rate.
- The apex beat is found on the left outermost and lowest point of the heart: the space between the left fifth and sixth ribs close to the midclavicular line.
- A weak rapid pulse is characteristic of shock.
- A cause of cardiogenic shock is myocardial infarction (MI); an area of dead or dying myocardium (the infarct) results from occlusion of the coronary arteries.
- The ECG P wave occurs with depolarisation of the atria (atrial contraction), followed by the PQ interval as the impulse disappears down the bundle of His; the QRS complex is depolarisation of the ventricles (ventricular contraction, or systole) followed by ventricular repolarisation, the T wave (ventricular relaxation).
- Sinus rhythm is a normal ECG pattern; arrhythmias are abnormal deviations from the ECG pattern.
- Valvular disorders create turbulence in the blood flow through the valve causing extra sounds (murmurs), e.g. stenosis, a narrowing of the valve opening, or incompetence, when a valve will not close properly.
- Bradycardia, confusion, nausea and coupled beats are signs of digoxin toxicity, and nurses should check the patients pulse before administration of this drug.
- The heart rate falls in children from 110–160 per minute below 1 year of age to 60–100 per minute over 12 years old.
- The brachial or temporal pulse should normally be used for younger children and the radial pulse should be used for older children; the carotid pulse should not be used in children.

References

Hatchett R., Arundale K. and Francis-Reme L. (1999) Systems and diseases: the heart, part four: basic cardiac arrhythmias. *Nursing Times*, 95(43): 44–47.

Levick J. R. (1992) *An Introduction to Cardiovascular Physiology*. Butterworth- Heinemann Ltd., Oxford.

Gordon K. and Child A. (2000a) Systems and diseases: The heart, part 9: heart failure 1. *Nursing Times*, 96(12): 53–56.

Gordon K. and Child A. (2000b) Systems and diseases: The heart, part 10: heart failure 2. *Nursing Times*, 96(16): 49–52.

Vickers J. (1999a) Systems and diseases: the heart, part one: anatomy and physiology. *Nursing Times*, 95(30): 42–45.

Vickers J. (1999b) Systems and diseases: the heart, part two: anatomy and physiology. *Nursing Times*, 95(34): 46–49.

Vickers J. (1999c) Systems and diseases: the heart, part three: anatomy and physiology. *Nursing Times*, 95(39): 46–49.

Chapter 3

Cardiovascular observations (II): blood pressure

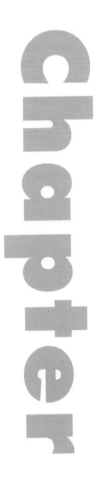

- Introduction
- Physiology of blood pressure
- Observations of blood pressure
- Drugs affecting the blood pressure
- Blood pressure in children
- Key points

Introduction

One of the problems of adopting an upright posture is the fact that the brain is then placed somewhat higher than the heart. This then requires the heart to sustain sufficient pressure of blood to supply the brain *uphill*, i.e. *against* gravity. Failure to do this would starve the brain of the vital glucose and oxygen it needs for consciousness and mental function. However, blood pressure is fundamental to the perfusion of blood through *all* the body tissues. Good examples are the kidneys, which must have adequate blood pressure to maintain filtration of urine, the lungs, which need a constant flow of blood for gas exchange, and the digestive system, which has a blood flow to collect nutrients from the diet. Any transport system must move, and movement of a fluid requires pressure. Blood pressure is an index of some of the most fundamental physiological processes in the body, and an understanding of arterial blood pressure and its measurement is essential for the accurate determination of physiological processes and disturbances.

Physiology of blood pressure

The systemic arterial **blood pressure** (**BP**) is caused *partly* by the contraction of the left ventricle. During **systole** (= ventricular contraction), the left ventricular myocardium pushes the **stroke volume** (**SV**) of blood into the aorta, and this surge of blood causes the aorta to stretch wider. The stroke volume, the amount of blood ejected with each ventricular contraction, is about 70 ml of blood per ventricle. The wave of high pressure generated continues through the arterial system causing the **systolic BP**, having an average peak of about 120 mmHg (millimetres of mercury) in the major systemic arteries in adults. This pressure falls as blood is distributed through the remaining arterial system and capillary bed, reaching its lowest at close to 0 mmHg in the venous return to the heart (Figure 3.1). During systole, the left ventricle is relaxing and filling with blood. There is no output to the aorta, and this creates a lower pressure in the systemic arteries, a **diastolic BP** of about 80–90 mmHg. The human BP in the major systemic arteries is therefore recorded as 120 over 90 mmHg. But if the left ventricle has no output during diastole, the diastolic pressure should *theoretically* fall to zero. Zero pressure would mean that blood flow has stopped, and this would be disastrous for the brain, which demands a constant blood supply (for oxygen and glucose). Without this supply the brain becomes unconscious (i.e. fainting). The heart goes through about 72 systoles

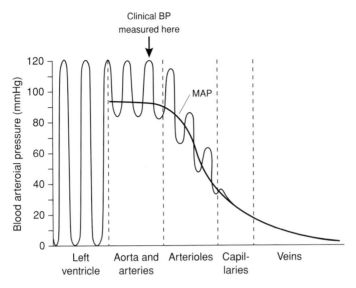

FIGURE 3.1 Blood pressure values through the arterial system. The left ventricle drops to 0 mmHg during diastole, the arterial diastolic pressure is maintained at about 80 mmHg in the arteries. Through the arterioles the mean arterial pressure (MAP) and both the systolic and the diastolic pressures drop with closure of the pulse pressure, i.e. a loss of the pulsatile nature of the flow by the capillaries.

and diastoles per minute, so at a *theoretical* systemic blood pressure of 120 over 0 mmHg, the person would *faint 72 times per minute*. Clearly this is not the case; therefore, diastolic pressure must be maintained sufficiently to supply the brain (and all the other tissues) during this period of zero cardiac output. To see how this is achieved, go back to the point where the *surge of blood causes the aorta to stretch wider* (p. 48). What stretches during systole must recoil during diastole, and it is this *aortic recoil* that continues to push blood onward to the tissues while the heart relaxes and refills (Figure 3.2). The aorta is effectively a *diastolic pump*, keeping the pressure up during this time. The same occurs with the pulmonary artery from the right side of the heart, where pulmonary recoil continues to push blood through the lungs during right ventricular diastole. However, since the pulmonary circulation is entirely contained within the chest cavity, the pressures within this circulation are not available for standard clinical observation. They are measured only during specialised invasive cardiac procedures.

In the first sentence of this BP section the word *partly* was used because the contraction of the left ventricle is not the entire story. Any pressure of a fluid in a tube is dependent on events taking place at *both*

Aortic output
120 mmHg

Aortic output
80 mmHg

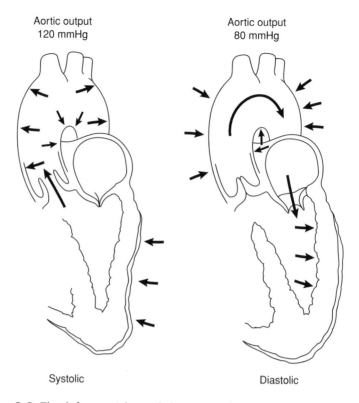

Systolic

Diastolic

FIGURE 3.2 The left ventricle and the aorta during the cardiac cycle. The short arrows indicate the direction of wall movement; the long arrows show the direction of blood flow. During systole, ventricular contraction occurs causing a high blood pressure resulting in aortic expansion. The aortic valve is open and the bicuspid valve is closed. In diastole the events are reversed, with the aortic recoil preventing the blood pressure from falling too low.

ends of that tube, i.e. the volume and force of the fluid entering the tube at one end (e.g. the cardiac output) and resistance to the flow of that fluid at the other end (e.g. the **peripheral resistance**, or **PR**). Take a garden hose as an example. The water enters the hose at one end from a tap and leaves at the other end. The output from the tap is the equivalent to the cardiac output. Although the output from the hose at the other end is sufficient to reach the nearby plants, those at the back of the flower bed may need a higher pressure to enable the water to reach them. This could be achieved by increasing the output from the tap, but it would probably be easier by placing a thumb over the end to narrow the opening and therefore increase the water pressure inside the tube. Water leaving the narrower opening does so at a higher pressure and therefore travels further. Removal of the thumb causes the water pressure to drop and therefore the jet of water returns to normal. In our garden hose the thumb acts as a peripheral resistance, and in the body the arterial peripheral resistance is achieved first by the reduction in size of the **arterioles** into a network of smaller vessels, and then by the **vasoconstriction** or **vasodilatation** that these smaller arterioles can achieve. In vasodilatation, the arteriole lumen widens and the peripheral resistance is *decreased* (like the thumb *removed* from the hose end), allowing the blood pressure to fall. In vasoconstriction, the arteriole lumen narrows and the peripheral resistance is *increased* (like the thumb *placed over* the hose end), forcing the blood pressure up (Figure 3.3). Involuntary smooth muscle in the arteriole wall makes the changes to the lumen in response to the **sympathetic nervous system**. This system is influenced by the **vasomotor centre (VMC)**, a series of diffuse nuclei in the medulla that has a profound effect on blood pressure (Figure 3.3). The VMC can initiate variations in the peripheral resistance by adjusting the sympathetic vasoconstrictor tone, the state of constriction of the smooth muscle wall affecting the lumen of the arterioles. Changes are made in this tone in response to fluctuations in the blood pressure, keeping the BP within normal limits

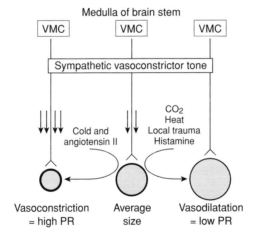

FIGURE 3.3 The vasomotor centre (VMC) and the local factors influencing the peripheral resistance (PR). Vasoconstriction is achieved by increasing the vasoconstrictor tone output from the VMC to the arterioles, or by the local action of cold or angiotensin II, causing the lumen to narrow and raising the PR. Vasodilatation is achieved by decreasing the sympathetic vasoconstrictor tone from the VMC or by the local action of heat, trauma, carbon dioxide or histamine, causing the lumen to widen and lowering of the PR. The number of arrows represents the strength of sympathetic stimulation.

for that individual. To do this the VMC must have feedback on what the pressure is, and this is achieved via **baroreceptors**, pressure-sensitive receptors found in the aortic arch and carotid arteries that directly measure the arterial BP and send this information to the VMC (Figure 3.4). When the BP is high, increased baroreceptor activity shuts down the VMC (i.e. **inhibition**), causing vasodilatation of the arterioles to lower the pressure. When the BP is low, decreased baroreceptor activity causes increased VMC output, which vasoconstricts the arterioles to raise the pressure. The VMC also responds to other factors and adjusts the BP accordingly. A lack of oxygen, an increase in carbon dioxide, mild pain, stress and increased chemoreceptor activity all cause more VMC activity and therefore vasoconstriction, raising the BP. Low carbon dioxide, severe pain and emotional shock all cause less VMC activity and therefore vasodilatation, lowering the BP (Figure 3.5). A sudden drop in the blood pressure is a not uncommon cause of fainting after a sudden emotional shock, such as bad news. Normal BP is maintained by an average vasoconstrictor tone stimulation from the VMC. Local factors influencing the peripheral resistance include cold, causing local vasoconstriction in the affected part, and heat, which will dilate the vessels. **Angiotensin II**, a vasoconstrictive hormone, has much wider effects on increasing the peripheral resistance and therefore also the blood pressure. Angiotensin II is activated under the emergency

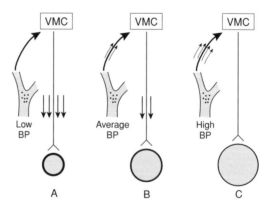

FIGURE 3.4 The effect of the baroreceptors on the VMC. A, in low blood pressure situations a lack of baroreceptor stimulation allows the VMC to cause vasoconstriction and this raises the blood pressure; B, average baroreceptor stimulation allows for normal peripheral resistance; C, high blood pressure causes considerable baroreceptor stimulation which inhibits the VMC output and causes vasodilatation to lower the blood pressure. The number of arrows in each case represents the degree of stimulation.

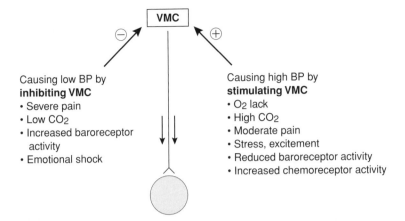

FIGURE 3.5 The factors affecting the VMC. Severe pain, low carbon dioxide, increased baroreceptor stimulation and emotional shock all inhibit the VMC and cause low blood pressure by vasodilatation. A lack of oxygen, high carbon dioxide, moderate pain, stress and excitement, reduced baroreceptor stimulation and increased chemoreceptor stimulation all stimulate the VMC causing higher blood pressure by vasoconstriction.

situation of low blood pressure to the kidneys (Figure 3.6), since blood pressure into the kidneys must be maintained to ensure that filtration continues (see Chapter 5). The metabolic wastes (**metabolites**) of muscle activity, such as **carbon dioxide** (see Figure 1.1), and chemical substances associated with **inflammation**, such as **histamine**, cause vasodilatation locally. So also does local **trauma** (injury), especially damage to the skin, as seen in **burns**.

Blood pressure can be seen as a *combination* of many effects; the output from the heart (the cardiac output, or CO = heart rate × stroke volume) at the front end of the tube, and the total peripheral resistance (PR) at the distal end of the tube. Thus

$$BP = CO \times PR \quad \text{or} \quad (HR \times SV) \times PR$$

Other effects involved include the viscosity (or thickness) of blood, which will vary according to the amount of water obtained from drinking or lost in the urine, and the elasticity of the vessel wall, which will stretch and recoil with the wave of pressure. Reduced elasticity, as seen with increasing age, will resist the pressure wave, which will then remain higher as a result, and if this is a feature throughout the vascular bed, the BP will remain higher than expected (see p. 60).

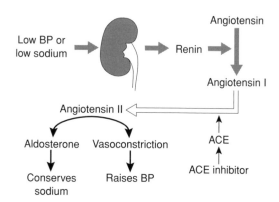

FIGURE 3.6 The renin–angiotensin–aldosterone cycle. Low blood pressure or low blood sodium causes the kidney to release renin. Renin activates angiotensin to angiotensin I, which is then further converted to angiotensin II by the angiotensin-converting enzyme (ACE). ACE function can be blocked by the ACE inhibitor drugs. Angiotensin II stimulates aldosterone secretion (to conserve sodium) and vasoconstriction (to raise blood pressure), thus correcting the original problem.

The difference between the systolic and diastolic pressures is called the **pulse pressure**, and it is about 30–40 mmHg in the aorta:

Pulse pressure = systolic pressure – diastolic pressure, e.g. $120 - 90$ = 30 mmHg.

The rapid narrowing and disappearance of the pulse pressure through the arterioles results in a loss of pulsation in the capillary network within the tissues, and therefore blood flows through the tissues continuously (known as **tissue perfusion**). The **mean arterial pressure (MAP)** is the main BP driving force of tissue perfusion. The MAP is influenced by both the cardiac output and the total peripheral resistance, which are themselves influenced by other factors (Figure 3.7). MAP is calculated by adding one-third of the pulse pressure to the diastolic pressure:

MAP = diastolic pressure + one-third pulse pressure, or
MAP = (systolic pressure – diastolic pressure) ÷ 3 + diastolic pressure,

and given our standard BP of 120 over 90 mmHg, the MAP would be

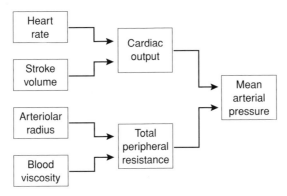

Figure 3.7 Factors contributing to the mean arterial pressure (MAP). The cardiac output and the total peripheral resistance are themselves influenced by other factors. The heart rate and stroke volume determine the cardiac output, and the anterior radius and blood viscosity determine the total peripheral resistance.

$$(120 - 90) \div 3 + 90 \quad \text{or} \quad 30 \div 3 + 90, \text{ i.e. } 10 + 90$$

which is 100 mmHg.

Since the heart is in the diastolic period of the cardiac cycle for longer than the systolic period (diastolic = 0.5 seconds, systolic = 0.3 seconds), the mean (= average) arterial pressure must be *closer* to the diastolic pressure, i.e. it is *not* simply the sum of the systolic pressure (SP) and diastolic pressure (DP) halved [i.e. (SP + DP) ÷ 2] as might be expected for an average. The MAP must be closely regulated because if it is too low the tissues would be deprived of a blood supply, and if it is too high it would cause vascular damage thereby increasing the work load of the heart.

Observations of blood pressure

Blood pressure measurement

The standard clinical blood pressure is measured in systemic arteries (i.e. from the left ventricle), usually the **brachial artery** running down the upper arm using a sphygmomanometer (sphygmo = pulse, manometer = pressure measure: the *pulse pressure measure*). The sphygmomanometer is used in conjunction with the **stethoscope**, through which the nurse will hear the sounds (= **auscultation**) associated with pressure changes as they occur in the artery. However, nothing is heard if a stethoscope is simply placed over an artery . This is because blood normally passes down arteries in a straight flow without any disturbance, and this movement is silent. It is generally considered that to create sounds that can be heard through a stethoscope, some disturbance to this blood flow is necessary, causing turbulence. Disturbance causes extra currents, so called **eddy currents**, and these disrupt the straightforward flow and cause sounds. To do this the artery has to be compressed sufficiently to reduce the lumen; this is a job for the sphygmomanometer.

It is important to carry out the procedure accurately to avoid false high or low readings as indicated in Table 3.1. The patient should be lying or seated comfortably with legs uncrossed and should not have changed position for 5 minutes before the procedure. The brachial artery at the point of the **antecubital fossa** (i.e. the *inside* of the elbow) of the patient's right arm should be level with the heart, supported on pillows on a firm surface to relax muscle tension, which may cause a false reading. The left arm should only be used if the right is unavailable, as would be the case if the right had been injured or had been used for an intravenous infusion. A small difference of 5–10 mmHg often exists between the left and right arms of the same individual, and choosing the right arm whenever possible ensures consistency each time the BP is taken. The brachial region above the elbow is exposed with no clothing restrictions above this. A cuff of the correct dimensions is placed around the upper arm *over* the brachial artery. The air bladder

TABLE 3.1 Blood pressure measurement errors

Error in technique	False high reading	False low reading
Artery below heart level	✓	
Artery above heart level		✓
Cuff too long		✓
Cuff too short	✓	
Cuff too narrow	✓	
No systolic estimation		✓
Overinflation of cuff	✓	
Deflation too slow	✓	
Deflation too fast		✓
Re-inflation without rest	✓	
Crossed legs	✓	
Unsupported arm	✓	
Tight clothing on upper arm	✓	

of the cuff should cover about two-thirds of the length of the upper arm and at least 80% of the arm circumference (recommended adult width of the bladder is 12–14 cm and the length is 35 cm). Too short an air bladder is more problematic than too long. The centre of the bladder should be in line with the brachial artery which would be located by palpation (= felt) at the anticubital fossa (Figure 3.8). As the cuff fills with air it compresses the arm, and therefore the artery, and the normal flow is disrupted as blood tries to pass the restriction. Sufficient cuff compression causes eddy currents to begin and the sound of blood flow can be heard in five phases (Korotkoff sounds, Table 3.2) through a stethoscope. The procedure is as follows:

Step 1: The systolic pressure should first be *estimated*, which is achieved by palpation of the brachial pulse during the *rapid* inflation of the cuff until the pulse can no longer be felt. Then, the *slow* deflation of the cuff allows the point to be noted where the brachial pulse returns, followed by rapid complete cuff deflation.

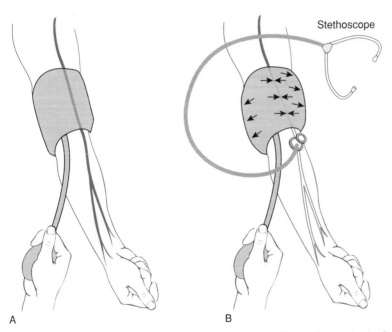

A   B

FIGURE 3.8 Right arm with sphygmomanometer cuff in place. A, before inflation of the cuff the artery is fully open and filled with blood (black); B, after inflation of the cuff the artery is compressed and empty of blood below the compression (i.e. inflated above systolic pressure). No sounds are heard through the stethoscope.

Estimation of the systolic pressure prevents overinflation of the cuff and allows the nurse to miss the **auscultatory gap**, a quiet period (Korotkoff phase II, Table 3.2) occurring between the systolic and diastolic points. If the cuff was inflated to an arbitrary point on the scale the nurse may then be listening to this gap, which could then be mistaken to be *above* the systolic, and a grossly false systolic pressure would be recorded.

Step 2: One minute is allowed before the full procedure continues; during this time the arm should be momentarily raised above the head to allow maximum drainage of the venous blood.

Step 3: Inflate the cuff to about 30 mmHg above the estimated systolic pressure, the inflation should be rapid to avoid excessive venous congestion.

Step 4: Deflate the cuff slowly, i.e. the recommended deflation rate is about 3 mmHg per second, or per heart beat if the pulse rate is 60 per minute. This rate accommodates most heart rates and prevents venous congestion in the distal vascular bed. During deflation the nurse is listening for the sounds through the stethoscope placed over the brachial artery just distal to, i.e. below, the cuff constriction. Above the systolic there is silence since the artery is fully compressed and all blood flow has stopped. Between the systolic down to the diastolic the sounds of 'thud, thud…' with each beat of the heart can be heard. From the diastolic down to 0 mmHg there is silence again (Figure 3.9). While deflating the cuff identify the start of the sounds (the upper point where sound begins, i.e. Korotkoff phase I) and mentally note this point as the systolic pressure. Continue to deflate slowly until the sounds disappear (in adults this is

TABLE 3.2 Korotkoff sounds and phases

Phase	Sounds
I	The appearance of faint, clear tapping sounds that gradually increase in intensity
II	The softening of sounds that may become swishing (possible auscultatory gap here)
III	The return of sharper sounds that become crisper but never fully regain the intensity of phase I
IV	The distinct abrupt muffling of sounds which become soft and blowing
V	The point at which all sounds cease

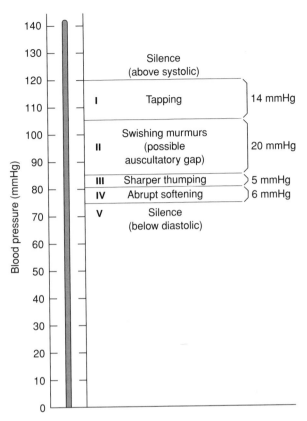

FIGURE 3.9 Korotkoff phases and sounds set against the mercury column (left) with the pressure differences between the phases shown (right).

Korotkoff phase V) and mentally note this point as the diastolic pressure, then fully deflate the cuff. Obviously do not keep the cuff inflated too long, especially above systolic pressure, since this cuts off all blood supply to the arm.

Step 5: If the procedure is to be repeated, a brief pause between attempts is necessary to allow blood to flow to and from the arm. Never re-inflate the cuff during or immediately after an attempt as this causes venous congestion and gives a false reading.

It is important to perfect the correct technique, including keeping the arm straight and supported, to maintain accuracy (Campbell *et al.* 1994). Although the sphygmomanometer is measuring the blood pressure, the process is *indirect.* The sphygmomanometer actually measures the pressure of the air in the cuff, but the nurse has skilfully arranged for this air pressure to exactly equal the blood pressure in the artery, first at systolic pressure and then at diastolic pressure.

Abnormal blood pressures

Abnormalities of systemic blood pressure means either the pressure is too high (**hypertension**) or too low (**hypotension**). In general, a guide to what is high or low is the pressure 100 mmHg. If the *diastolic* goes *above* 100 mmHg this suggests hypertension, but if the *systolic* goes *below* 100 mmHg this suggests hypotension.

Blood pressure rises gradually with age normally, but hypertension produces symptoms resulting from damage to organs and tissues, especially the heart itself and the blood vessels. **Essential hypertension** appears to have no identifiable cause, but whatever the cause is it results in sodium and water retention which drives the BP up. **Secondary hypertension** follows on from another pathology, particularly chronic renal disease, which may be accompanied by renin release (see renin–angiotensin–aldosterone cycle, p. 54) or tumours of the adrenal or pituitary glands. **Malignant hypertension** is regarded as a *diastolic* pressure exceeding 130 mmHg. It may be irreversible and can cause renal injury leading to kidney failure and death within a few years. The result of persistent hypertension can be any combination of three **complications**:

1 **cardiac hypertrophy**, or enlargement of the heart, leading ultimately to heart failure (**congestive cardiac failure**, or **CCF**);
2 **arteriosclerosis**, or *hardening of the arteries* due to blood vessel wall changes (which themselves will aggravate the high BP problem); and
3 **cerebrovascular accidents** (**CVAs**) (see 'Strokes', Chapter 7).

The risk of developing hypertension is increased as a result of:

1 being male (women suffer less)
2 increasing age
3 obesity
4 high levels of salt in the diet
5 smoking (nicotine is a vasoconstrictor) and sometimes
6 a family history of high blood pressure.

It is interesting that 50% of these risk factors are controllable by the individual, meaning that everyone has the opportunity to significantly reduce their risk of hypertension by losing weight, not smoking and reducing salt intake.

Low blood pressure is strongly resisted in the body by **compensatory mechanisms** which drive the BP up. Rapid compensation to increase BP quickly involves the vasoconstriction of distal arterioles to increase the total peripheral resistance, mediated through the sympathetic vasomotor tone and local factors (Figure 3.5), plus increases in heart rate and stroke volume to improve the cardiac output, mediated through sympathetic influences and some hormones, notably **adrenaline** (from the adrenal medulla) and **thyroid hormone** (from the thyroid gland). **Noradrenaline** has the action of selective vasoconstriction (e.g. in the skin), which will increase the PR, and also acts by increasing the **venomotor tone**, which causes a tightening of the veins to improve the venous return of blood to the heart. **Cortisol** is another important hormone that helps in the compensatory mechanisms by preventing water from leaving the circulation into the tissues, thus helping to stabilise the blood volume. Cortisol reduces the permeability of the capillary wall to water and is secreted in higher volumes than normal from the adrenal cortex during stress. In the slightly longer term, water conservation to boost blood volume, and therefore increase BP, can be achieved through greater secretion of **antidiuretic hormone** (**ADH**, from the hypothalamus via the posterior pituitary). ADH conserves water directly by acting on the distal half of the renal tubule. In addition, sodium conservation by **aldosterone** (from the adrenal cortex) by also acting on the distal renal tubule has the effect of conserving water indirectly.

Postural hypotension, a drop in blood pressure on changing position from lying to sitting up or standing, is expected in everyone to some extent, but rapid compensatory adjustments ensure that for most people it is not a problem. It can become a difficulty experienced with increasing age, and nurses should be aware of this when moving elderly people from one position to another. Getting them up from the bed onto a chair, or from the chair to standing, should be done *slowly* and in stages, allowing time for the BP to adjust after each stage. Communication with the patient is of key importance, allowing the patient to decide the pace of the move and when to rest, and to give the patient the chance to signal any symptoms of low BP that may be experienced, such as feeling faint or dizzy. **Post-operative observations** are critical to the patient's full recovery, and BP checks are paramount among these. Low blood pressure after surgery may indicate blood loss is occurring, either internally or externally, and should be reported and acted on quickly.

The ultimate extreme of profound hypotension occurs as a feature of **shock**, and this represents a stage where the compensatory mechanisms have failed to maintain the BP. Both the stroke volume and the cardiac output fall and therefore so does the blood pressure. Hypovolaemic shock results from **haemorrhage** (haemo = blood, rrhage = bursts forth), which may be internal (within body cavities, or as **bruising** into tissues) or external (into the outside environment). It is difficult to think of bruising as a potential cause of shock, but on an extensive scale it constitutes a considerable amount of blood lost from circulation. At risk of severe shock from bruising are elderly people after a fall downstairs or a brutal assault. Bleeding can be either arterial, venous or capillary. Arterial is far more serious as blood is lost from a high-pressure system in pulses, and speed is essential to control this before the person exsanguinates (bleeds to death).

Other forms of shock occur even when the blood volume remains normal. These are:

1 **cardiogenic shock**, when the heart as a pump fails to sustain a normal stroke volume; and
2 **vasogenic shock**, where the cause is the vascular system itself.

A common cause of cardiogenic shock is **myocardial infarction (MI)**, where an area of *dead or dying myocardium* (= the infarct) results from occlusion of the coronary arteries. If this occurs in the ventricular myocardium the force of contraction, and therefore the stroke volume and blood pressure, is greatly reduced.

Vasogenic shock includes several forms depending on the cause. **Neurogenic shock** occurs when the sympathetic nervous system supply to the cardiovascular system is blocked causing a low cardiac output, reduced peripheral resistance and venous blood pooling. Venous pooling is an important cause of lost circulating blood volume since the veins carry the majority of the blood volume in circulation at any given time, and when this fails to return to the heart it produces a poor cardiac output. **Anaphylactic shock** is due to a severe allergic reaction, resulting in massive release of the inflammatory chemical **histamine** (see histamine, p. 53), which causes a rapid body-wide vasodilatation with profound loss of peripheral resistance and collapse of the blood pressure.

Apart from hypotension and tachycardia, shock, whatever the type, will also cause collapse of the individual affected and altered consciousness (e.g. fainting) as the blood supply to the brain is reduced.

Other symptoms include pallor (pale skin colour) and cold skin, caused by diversion of blood away from the skin to the vital organs (see noradrenaline, p. 61), and sweating, caused by sympathetic stimulation of the sweat glands, a side-effect of the sympathetic compensatory mechanism.

Drugs affecting the blood pressure

Since many cardiac drugs have an effect on both the pulse and the blood pressure, much of the information on these drugs has been given in Chapter 2. Some drugs act to raise the blood pressure but others serve to lower it.

Positive inotropic drugs are those that increase the force of contraction and by raising the cardiac output they increase the blood pressure. These include the **cardiac glycosides** (e.g. **digoxin**) and the **phosphodiesterase inhibitors** (see Chapter 2 for details).

Drugs required to lower the BP as a treatment of hypertension include the **angiotensin-converting enzyme inhibitors (ACE inhibitors)** (see Chapter 2), which reduce the blood pressure by preventing the formation of angiotensin II, blocking its vasoconstrictive effects (Figure 3.6). The result is a reduction in peripheral resistance, and thus a drop in blood pressure. Beta-blocking drugs also provide an decrease in the cardiac output and a lower BP (see Chapter 2 and Figure 3.10).

The **diuretics** make up a group of drugs that lower the BP (and are therefore used as a treatment in hypertension) by causing a larger urine output (see Chapter 5). They do this by inhibiting the re-absorption of sodium, mostly in the second convoluted tubule of the renal nephron. The extra sodium excreted as a result takes with it extra water, and this water loss reduces the blood volume, one of the influencing factors in BP maintenance. Some diuretic drugs may also have a vasodilatory effect *outside* the kidney, which has some part to play in lowering the BP.

Blood pressure in children

The systolic blood pressure rises normally with age, averaging at about 90 mmHg at 1 year old to about 100 mmHg at 12 years old, although great variation occurs according to growth rate and size. It is important when taking the child's blood pressure to use a cuff of the correct size for their age:

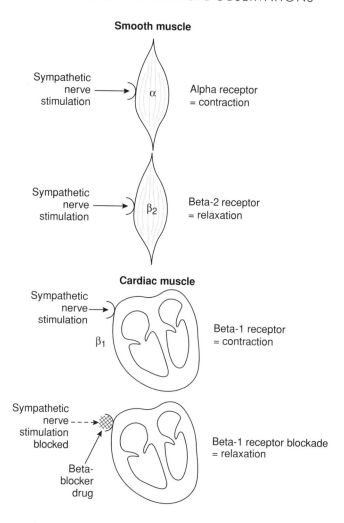

Figure 3.10 The action of beta-blocker drugs. Sympathetic stimulation of smooth muscles may cause contraction if the alpha (α) receptor is activated or relaxation if the beta-2 (β_2) receptor is activated. On cardiac muscle, sympathetic stimulation of the beta-1 (β_1) receptor causes the heart to increase the heart rate and force of contraction, unless the receptor is blocked by drugs that prevent sympathetic stimulation and the heart slows down and decreases the force of contraction. Beta-blocking drugs may cause side-effects by blocking beta-receptors on smooth muscle (e.g. causing broncho-constriction).

Age	Cuff width
Neonate	2–5 cm
1–4 years	6 cm
4–8 years	9 cm

The wrong size cuff, especially the use of an adult size cuff with children, will result in inaccurate results. The procedure also varies in children, with the Korotkoff stage IV sounds (Table 3.2) used to determine diastolic pressure. Children tend to have a higher cardiac output for body size than adults and this causes the fifth-phase Korotkoff sounds, used in adults for determining the diastolic pressure, to be too low for paediatric clinical use.

Key points

- Blood pressure = cardiac output × peripheral resistance (BP = CO × PR), where the CO = heart rate × stroke volume (CO = HR × SV).
- The average adult arterial BP is 120 systolic over 80 diastolic measured in mmHg (millimetres of mercury).
- The difference between the systolic and diastolic pressures is called the pulse pressure.
- The mean arterial pressure is calculated by adding one-third of the pulse pressure to the diastolic pressure, i.e. MAP = diastolic pressure + one-third pulse pressure.
- The systolic blood pressure rises normally with age, about 90 mmHg at 1 year old to about 100 mmHg at 12 years old; variation occurs according to growth rate and size.
- It is important to use a cuff that is the correct size for adults and correct for a child's age; the wrong size cuff will give inaccurate results.

References

Campbell N. R., McKay D. W., Chockalingam A. and Fodor J. G. 1994 Errors in assessment of blood pressure: blood pressure measuring technique. *Canadian Journal of Public Health*, 85(Suppl. 2): S18–21.

Chapter 4

Respiratory observations

- Introduction
- The respiratory physiology
- The neurophysiology of respiration
- Observations of breathing
- Childhood breathing

Introduction

We breathe because we need oxygen (O_2) from the air; although this is essentially true, oxygen is however not the main driving force of breathing. The primary driving force is carbon dioxide (CO_2), i.e. the need to remove this gas from the body. In Chapter 1 we identified how CO_2 was a by-product of energy production, a means of shedding surplus carbon from the body (see Figure 1.1). The excretory pathway of this gas is via the lungs, having first been transported there by the blood from the tissues. Nursing observations of respiration should be thought of as a means of assessing the efficiency of this process and detecting any abnormalities. Carbon dioxide is both beneficial and harmful, depending on the quantity present. Constant volumes of this gas in both the tissues and the blood are essential to maintain the driving force that keeps us breathing (and thus taking in oxygen), yet too much carbon dioxide will cause congestion of the biochemistry of energy production to the point where this would threaten the very existence of life itself. Compared with this, oxygen has a smaller role in maintaining the respiratory drive, although it is still important, and its complete absence is also incompatible with life.

Respiratory physiology

The **alveoli** of the lungs (minute air sacs that make up the bulk of lung tissue) provide the location for gas exchange between the blood and the atmosphere. There are three gas exchange compartments: the *air* within the alveoli (appropriately called **alveolar air**), the *blood* and the *tissues* of the alveolar wall (Figure 4.1). While the air and blood are constantly being changed, the tissues provide a constant close, yet distinct, barrier between the two. Movement of gases across this barrier uses a fundamental driving force: the **concentration gradient**. Gases, liquids and many elementary particles will flow from a point of high concentration to a point of low concentration if given the opportunity to do so, a movement referred to as **diffusion**. Diffusion is defined as the movement of **solutes** (substances dissolved in a solvent), gas or liquid particles from the point where their concentration is greatest to all other points of lower concentration. In the case of respiration, diffusion refers to the movement of the respiratory gases oxygen and carbon dioxide across the tissues between the alveoli and the blood. The object of diffusion is to equalise the concentrations at both points. However, in the lungs this equalisation is never achieved, which is just

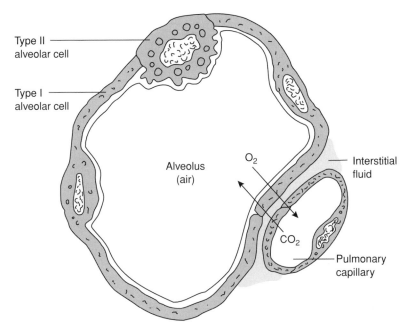

Figure 4.1 Microscopic view of the lung, showing an alveolus containing air, with walls of type I and type II cells, a pulmonary capillary containing blood, and interstitial fluid between the capillary and the alveolus. The direction of gas movement is shown.

as well since if it was the gases would stop flowing and we would die from respiratory failure (**asphyxiation**). At the same time a lack of oxygen, and carbon dioxide poisoning would occur in the tissues. During breathing, oxygen is normally moving into the blood, but is kept in higher concentrations in the lungs than in the blood by the continued addition of new oxygen from the air. Similarly, carbon dioxide is moving into the lungs, but the concentration of this gas in the lungs is kept lower than in the blood by the continued removal of carbon dioxide from the lungs by breathing. In this way, the act of breathing itself ensures that these concentration gradients are maintained and therefore these gases will continue to flow in and out of the lungs and blood.

That act of breathing is a mechanical process that involves the movement of muscles within the chest wall and diaphragm. Chest wall and diaphragmatic movements govern lung expansion and contraction because the lungs are held tightly against the chest wall by a slight negative pressure (or vacuum, i.e. minus 4 mmHg) which exists between a membrane attached to the outer surface of the lungs (the **visceral layer** of the **pleura**) and a membrane attached to the inner surface of the chest wall (the **parietal layer** of the pleura), causing these two surfaces to stay stuck close together (Figure 4.2). This suction force is created because the negative intrapleural pressure is 4 mmHg *lower* than the atmospheric pressure, which is both outside the chest wall and inside the lungs at rest. In this sense, it is useful to think of the lungs as being 'vacuum packed', like some foods sold at the supermarket. Whatever movements the chest wall makes the lungs must go along with it, unless the vacuum is broken by the introduction of an abnormal substance between the two pleural layers. If this substance is air, this causes a condition called **pneumothorax**; if it is water, the condition is called **hydrothorax**, the water being derived from blood; and if it is whole blood, the condition is called **haemothorax**. Any combination can exist, such as **haemopneumothorax**. In any of these cases the lung will fall away from the chest wall in varying degrees and fail to respond to chest wall movements, making breathing very difficult.

The muscle movements of the chest wall operate the ribs, which during inspiration are moved upwards and outwards, expanding the volume (or space) within the chest from front to back and side to side. Contraction of the diaphragm at the same time causes it to flatten, increasing the chest volume from top to bottom. The lungs are stretched

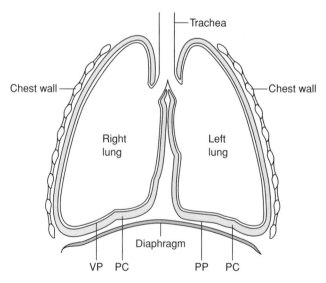

Figure 4.2 The lungs and the pleural membrane. PC, pleural cavity containing the negative (suction) pressure; PP, parietal layer of the pleural membrane attached to the chest wall and diaphragm; VP, visceral layer of the pleural membrane attached to the lung surface.

outwards in all directions, causing the air pressure inside the lungs to drop below atmospheric pressure, thus creating a partial vacuum within the lungs which must be instantly filled by air taken in from the atmosphere (**inhalation** or **inspiration**). The reverse is also true, when the respiratory muscles relax, allowing the ribs and diaphragm to return to their previous normal position. This squeezes the lungs, increasing the pressure inside the lungs above atmospheric pressure, which then forces the air back out into the atmosphere (**exhalation** or **expiration**) (Figure 4.3). The relationship between volume and pressure seen in the lungs is expressed in **Boyle's law**, where the pressure inside the lungs falls if the volume increases at a constant temperature (as in inhalation), or the pressure rises if the volume decreases at a constant temperature (as in exhalation). The muscles used during normal breathing are **primary**, since they act all the time. However, sometimes events require additional effort to be put into the breathing process, for example immediately after a fast race, and some extra **secondary** (or **accessory**) muscles are used to assist in chest wall movement. These standby muscles of breathing include some of the muscles of the neck and shoulder region. The most efficient position for the use of these muscles is upright, leaning slightly forward, with arms raised to a horizontal position. Severely breathless patients will adopt this position to aid their breathing if they are able to do so.

The volume of air we take in with each breath is the **tidal volume**, i.e. air moving in and out of the lungs like water moves with the tides. This volume is about 500 ml of air in adults, depending on the size variation that occurs between different adults. A closer look reveals, however, that this volume can be subdivided into two different volumes based on functional grounds, i.e. a volume which *will* reach the alveoli and exchange gas with the blood (the alveolar air) and the volume that *will not* reach the alveoli and thus does not exchange gas (called the **dead space**). Dead space air fills the air passages, the **trachea**, the **bronchi** and the **bronchioles**. Exhaled dead space air contains the same gas mixture as inhaled air, whereas alveolar air has more carbon dioxide and less oxygen in it due to exchange with the blood. So we can state a simple formula:

Tidal volume (TV) = alveolar air + dead space air

The dead space remains relatively constant, averaging about 150 ml of air (with some variation between individuals), unless there is any change

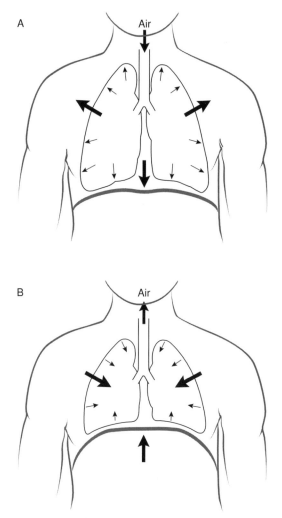

FIGURE 4.3 Inspiration and expiration. A, during inspiration the chest wall moves upwards and outwards, the diaphragm flattens causing the lungs to be stretched in all directions. The resulting increase in the volume inside the lungs causes the pressure to fall and air is drawn in to fill the space; B, during expiration the return of the lungs and diaphragm decreases the lung space forcing the pressure up and air is blown out.

in the diameter of the bronchi or the bronchioles, the only parts of the air passages capable of changing their diameter (known as bronchoconstriction if the diameter narrows or bronchodilation if the diameter widens). For most purposes, these changes can be ignored and calculations involving tidal volume assume a constant dead space. It therefore becomes easy to calculate the alveolar air volume: 500 ml (TV) – 150 ml (dead space) = 350 ml of alveolar air at rest. But these values change during exercise, when we breathe faster and harder. Exercise actually causes us to increase our tidal volume by stretching the lungs further than at rest. A bigger tidal volume means a bigger alveolar air volume rather than dead space volume since the air passages, and therefore the dead space, will increase less. Increases in the alveolar air volume provide more air available for gas exchange with the blood, and respiration becomes more efficient. But respiration also speeds up with exercise, and this can reduce the efficiency if the respiratory rate increases too much. The reason for this is that by squeezing more tidal volumes in per minute, each tidal volume has less time to get in and out, and this results in a smaller tidal volume with each breath taken. Again, assuming a relatively constant dead space, the largest reduction must occur in the alveolar air, making less air available for gas exchange and therefore reducing lung efficiency. Slow, *deep* breathing is more efficient than rapid *shallow* breathing. Here, the words deep and shallow reflect the size of the tidal volume: deep is a *large* tidal volume (mostly alveolar air = efficient) and shallow is a *small* tidal volume (mostly dead space = not efficient). The tidal volume is taken in and out about 18 times per minute at rest (the **respiratory rate** or **RR**). Multiplying the tidal volume with the respiratory rate will give the total volume of air moved in and out of the lungs per minute: the **pulmonary ventilation rate** (**PVR**; thus TV × RR = PVR). It may be important to calculate how much of the PVR is alveolar air, i.e. how much air is exchanging gases with the blood per minute (called the **alveolar ventilation rate**, or **AVR**). This is worked out by deducting the dead space from the tidal volume before multiplying that answer by the respiratory rate: i.e. (TV – dead space) × RR = AVR.

Some patients require a surgical procedure that shortens the airway, a **tracheostomy**, where they breathe through an opening in the throat, directly into the trachea below the larynx. A tracheostomy tube is often in place to maintain the opening. This procedure is done either to relieve, or by-pass an obstruction, or to reduce the dead space in those who will be ventilated for some time, thus making ventilation more efficient. Nurses should always check that breathing is normal through a tracheostomy and that no infection or obstruction occurs.

We have a functional **inspiratory reserve volume** (**IRV**), i.e. the maximum inspiration we can possibly take during a deep breath, and a functional **expiratory reserve volume** (**ERV**), i.e. the maximum expiration we can possibly produce by forced exhalation. The increase in tidal volume during exercise is in fact a widening of the TV into both the IRV and ERV volumes (Figure 4.4). In other words, we breathe deeper during exercise by using up some of our inspiratory and expiratory reserve volumes and adding it to our tidal volume. All the potentially expellable air volumes in the lungs add up to create the **vital capacity (VC)**, i.e. VC = IRV + ERV + TV. The vital capacity can be measured using an instrument called the **spirometer** or the **vitalograph**, which is a portable spirometer. Both require the subject to take a maximum inspiration, followed by a forced maximum expiration into a tube attached to the machine; the output is recorded on a chart. A **forced expiratory volume** in 1 second (**FEV$_1$**) can be directly measured, i.e. the amount of air that can be forcefully expired in 1 second after maximum inspiration. The use of a constant time period (1 second) enables standardisation between subjects. Most individuals will normally expire about 80% of their vital capacity in 1 second, but reduced patency of the airway (e.g. as in asthma) will delay this process, and the total vital capacity will take several seconds more to expire.

We can never breathe out all the air in our lungs, to do so would require the lungs to collapse; this remaining volume is called the

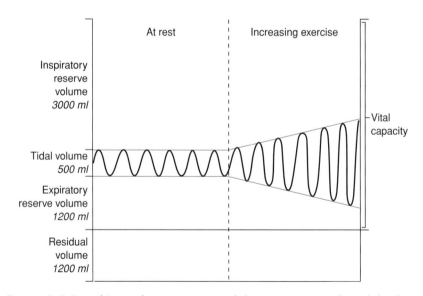

Figure 4.4 Breathing volumes at rest and during exercise. The tidal volume (TV) is approximately 500 ml at rest. As exercise begins the TV increases by incorporating part of the lungs' inspiratory reserve volume (IRV) and expiratory reserve volume (ERV). The residual volume remains in the lungs preventing lung collapse. The vital capacity (VC) represents the entire movable air in or out of the lungs and is the sum of IRV + ERV + TV.

residual volume. The residual volume still exchanges gas with the atmosphere and with the blood. Although it is a volume that remains constant in the lungs, that volume is being replaced by new air all the time.

The neurophysiology of respiration

The control of respiration is dependent on the respiratory centre, a collection of several neuronal groups shared between the **medulla** and the **pons**, both parts of the **brain stem**. The respiratory centre not only makes us breathe by sending nerve impulses to the muscles of the respiratory mechanism but also increases the respiratory rate and depth as required. There are many factors that influence the respiratory centre, but, as we have seen, the most important of these is the CO_2 level in the blood. Rising CO_2 blood level stimulates the centre to increase the rate and depth of breathing, with the effect of increasing the excretion of CO_2, whereas a low CO_2 blood level shuts down the stimulus on the respiratory centre and breathing becomes slow and shallow in order to retain CO_2. Complete absence of CO_2 in the blood would cause **apnoea**, i.e. complete cessation of breathing, simply because this would remove any incentive to breathe. This is a typical feedback mechanism, part of the body's homeostatic status designed to regulate the internal environment within defined parameters, in this case the blood gas concentrations. **Chemoreceptors** in the carotid and aortic arteries and in the medulla itself are sensory nerve endings specialising in detecting the gas composition of the blood and feeding this information back to the respiratory centre. These chemoreceptors are also sensitive to the pH of the blood, i.e. the acid–base balance of the plasma; pH is a measure of the hydrogen ion concentration ($[H^+]$), and a high H^+ concentration causes acidic conditions. Normally blood is about pH 7.4, just on the alkaline side of neutral (pH 7.0), and this blood pH level is critical. A change of just 0.1 in the pH can be hazardous to health. CO_2 is thought of as an acid gas because in combination with water (as in plasma) it forms carbonic acid ($CO_2 + H_2O = H_2CO_3$), and H_2CO_3 (carbonic acid) can liberate H^+ (i.e. $H_2CO_3 \rightarrow HCO_3^- + H^+$). For this reason, any CO_2 retention creates a **respiratory acidosis** of the blood. In such acidic conditions of the blood, high concentrations of H^+ (= low pH) can be corrected *in the short term* by stimulating respiration to excrete more CO_2, thus forming less carbonic acid. Alternatively, any oxygen lack mostly stimulates the carotid chemoreceptors, which will increase respiration to improve oxygen intake.

The respiratory centre has several separate groups of neurones, some in the medulla and some in the pons (Figure 4.5). The medullary **inspiratory centre**, called the **dorsal respiratory group** (**DRG**), sends nerve impulses to the muscles of respiration causing contraction of these muscles in an on–off cyclic pattern. Switching on causes inspiration, and switching off permits expiration, a passive event during rest that occurs when relaxed muscles allow the return of the chest wall to a natural position. The medullary **ventral respiratory group** (**VRG**) helps to maintain the muscle tone of the inspiratory muscles and also actively assists the chest wall expiratory muscles during forceful

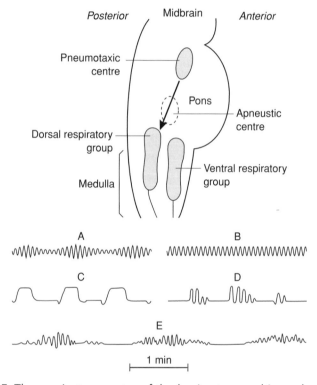

Figure 4.5 The respiratory centre of the brain stem and irregular forms of breathing. The dorsal respiratory group provides inspiratory signals at all times, and the ventral respiratory group helps to trigger inspiration during times of greater pulmonary need, e.g. exercise. The pneumotaxic centre of the pons influences the cut-off point for inspiration to prevent overinflation of the lungs. This cut-off signal may be itself blocked by the apneustic centre under various conditions, thus allowing increased inspiration. Abnormal forms of breathing are shown. A, Cheyne–Stokes; B, central neurogenic hyperventilation; C, apneustic breathing; D, cluster breathing; E, Biot's (ataxic) breathing (see text for explanation).

breathing, as in exercise, when passive expiration alone is not fast enough. The pons **pneumotaxic centre** sends inhibitory impulses to the DRG in order to limit inspiration and therefore fine tune the rhythm and prevent overinflation of the lungs. The function of the pons **apneustic centre** is less well understood. Impulses from this centre stimulate the DRG and would prolong inspiration if the DRG was not inhibited by the pneumotaxic centre. However, the apneustic centre itself can be directly inhibited by the pneumotaxic centre (Hickey 1997, see also Figure 4.5). Feedback to the DRG on inspiration comes also from the lungs themselves, via stretch receptors located in the bronchi and bronchioles throughout the lungs.

The medullary breathing centre has morphine receptors, i.e. cell surface proteins that bind drugs such as morphine. These are known as μ-receptors (pronounced 'mu'). Elsewhere in the medulla, morphine-like drugs binding to μ-receptors block pain. On the respiratory centre, however, morphine binding to these receptors causes respiratory depression, i.e. breathing will slow down and become shallow. Any patient receiving morphine for pain should be observed for shallow, slow breathing as a side-effect of the drug. In these cases it may prove detrimental to the patient, especially elderly people or those with chronic respiratory disease, and the drug should be reduced or replaced.

Abnormalities of the breathing pattern (Figure 4.5) are sometimes due to disturbances affecting the respiratory centre, e.g. after **head injury** or due to **raised intracranial pressure (RICP)**. **Cheyne–Stokes** respiration is a rhythmic coming and going (waxing and waning) of the depth and rate of breathing interspersed by periods of apnoea. The cycle occurs over about 1 minute, within which breathing stops for about 20 seconds. An increase in carbon dioxide sensitivity and decrease in stimulation from the respiratory centre results in this pattern of breathing. The lesion responsible is not clear; it is often bilateral, deep in the cerebral hemispheres or within the basal nuclei. **Apneustic breathing** refers to a prolonged inspiration of 2 or 3 seconds followed by a long expiratory pause. A complete respiratory cycle takes about 50 seconds, during which the patient has breathed once. The lesion responsible is within the pons area, often caused by a blockage (occlusion) of the main arterial blood supply in the area. **Cluster breathing** is the term used to describe a series of rapid breaths (five or six together) which diminish in depth to complete apnoea for 20 seconds or so before starting again. The lesion responsible is in the lower pons or upper medulla. **Biot's (ataxic) breathing** shows a random unpredictable breathing pattern with shallow and deep inspirations and periods of pause. The lesion is in the medulla. **Central neurogenic hyperventilation** is a continuous pattern of fast, deep breaths, caused by lesions probably in the midbrain or pontine area of the brain stem. Such rapid breathing causes **alkalosis** (raised blood pH level, i.e. above pH 7.4), since CO_2 is lost to excess, and clearly indicates that CO_2 stimulation of breathing is no longer the case (Hickey 1997).

Observations of breathing

Assessment of the respiratory system is critical to our understanding of the patient's oxygen delivery system to the tissues and of carbon dioxide excretion: the patient's cellular metabolism depends on both (Owen 1998).

Respiratory rate and depth

Respiratory rate, the number of breathing cycles per minute, is the usual respiratory observation made by nurses. As adults, we breathe on average about 12–18 times per minute, but the rate can climb to 30 or more as a result of exercise, which provides additional oxygen, or as a result of some respiratory and cardiovascular disorders. A breathing cycle consists of an inspiration, an expiration and a brief pause. Modest increases in respiratory rate and tidal volume improve respiratory efficiency, as we have noted happens in exercise. But too fast a rate is inefficient, and so too is a very slow rate, e.g. below 12 breaths per minute, unless there is a greater *depth* of breathing (i.e. increased TV). Fast respiratory rates (**tachypnoea**), i.e. up to 30 per minute, can also be seen in infections involving fever, especially respiratory infections. Fever involves increased breathing rates, probably to supply additional oxygen for the raised tissue metabolism caused by activation of the body's defences. Faster breathing may also help to cool the body (see Chapter 1) as panting does in dogs. **Hyperventilation** is overbreathing, which may be due to physical or psychological causes. Pain and stress can both cause hyperventilation, and it is a feature of emotional reactions such as panic. Hyperventilation itself can severely reduce the carbon dioxide levels in the blood, which would normally slow breathing down by taking away the main respiratory drive. However, the higher centres of the brain, i.e. those involved in the stress reaction, override this chemical stimulus and drive respiration independently of carbon dioxide levels. The carbon dioxide loss causes symptoms such as peripheral tingling and numbness, stiff contractions of the hands and fingers and a feeling of unreality; all of which may add to the patient's stress.

Normally, oxygen and carbon dioxide in the blood create between them a gas pressure (the **blood gas tensions**), rather like the pressure created by the gas in an unopened fizzy drink bottle. Each gas contributes part of this total pressure, and this is known as the partial pressure of oxygen (Po_2) or the partial pressure of carbon dioxide (Pco_2). They are not equal since they depend on the volume of each gas carried by the blood. The Po_2 of *arterial* blood is 13.3 kPa (kilopascals) (100 mmHg), whereas the Pco_2 is 5.3 kPa (40 mmHg). The values for *venous* blood reflect the loss of oxygen from the blood to the tissues and the gain of carbon dioxide from the tissues to the blood (venous Po_2 = 5.3 kPa or 40 mmHg; Pco_2 = 6.1 kPa or 46 mmHg, where 1 kPa = 7.5 mmHg) (Figure 4.6). Respiratory rate increases would therefore result from increased Pco_2 or decreased Po_2 in arterial blood. Accurate

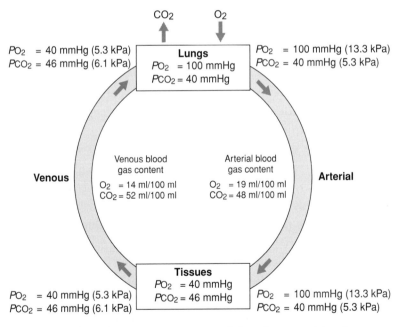

FIGURE 4.6 The blood gas tensions in arterial and venous blood compared with the gas tensions of the lungs and tissues. Notice that the arterial blood gas tensions adopt the same values as the lungs, and the venous blood gas tensions adopt the same values as the tissues (measured in mmHg and kPa). Blood gas contents are also shown for arterial and venous blood.

measurement of these values requires an *arterial* blood sample for analysis, since this records the results of gas exchange events taking place in the lungs (i.e. one of several lung function tests). A venous blood sample analysis would only reflect gas exchange in the tissues, and this is not useful for the diagnosis of lung disease. **Dyspnoea** means difficulty in breathing, and is recognised by the patient becoming very anxious and struggling to breathe (**air hunger**) including attempts to sit upright and forward if possible (see p. 71), a rapid respiratory rate, cyanosis (see p. 85) and possibly various abnormal respiratory sounds (Grey 1995) (see p. 84). Fast intervention is needed to relieve both the lack of oxygen and the distress caused by dyspnoea, depending on the cause. Difficulty in breathing can occur in air containing less oxygen than required (**rarefied air**), as noted at high altitudes in those not acclimatised to the situation. Not only is there less oxygen, but the altitude also involves lower air pressure, which exacerbates the problem. Deep-sea diving can also cause problems, because the increased water pressure on the body with depth allows more gas to be carried in the blood, additional gas that must be removed *slowly* (by decompression) as the diver comes to the surface. Failure to do this results in rapid release of the extra gas into the circulation, forming gas bubbles in the blood (**gas emboli**, a condition known as **the bends**), which can cause the death of the diver.

Patients may often experience difficulty in breathing while lying flat (known as **orthopnoea**), which necessitates their sleeping in an upright position. The sitting-up position improves breathing because it allows for greater chest expansion (no restriction of chest wall movement caused by the bed) and improves the flattening of the diaphragm (gravity removes the pressure caused by the abdominal contents below). In addition, any fluids in the lungs drain by gravity towards the base while sitting up, freeing the apical areas of the lungs, which have a better blood supply and are therefore more efficient for gas exchange.

In respiratory and heart diseases, the cause of an increased respiratory rate is a lack of oxygen (low Po_2), which the increased rate attempts to rectify. **Obstructive respiratory** (or **pulmonary**) **diseases** include **asthma**, where bronchoconstriction and mucosal swelling narrow the airway; **bronchitis**, where chronic swollen mucous membrane with excessive secretions obstruct the airway; and **emphysema**, where breakdown of the alveolar wall reduces the surface available for gas exchange. **Chronic bronchitis** is a disease associated with a cold, wet climate and smoking. Over many years, the reduced gas exchange commonly identified in this disease causes persistently reduced oxygen (low Po_2) in the blood. The respiratory centre normally responds to **hypoxia** (low O_2) by stimulating breathing. In diseased and inefficient lungs CO_2 can be retained, and the patient becomes reliant on the hypoxia to maintain breathing. Consequently, when the patient is admitted, nurses should not initiate oxygen therapy without medical advice, since the correction of the hypoxia may decrease the respiratory drive, worsen the lung efficiency and increase the retained CO_2. The result could be a respiratory acidosis. Oxygen may seem the obvious treatment for the breathless, cyanosed patient, but under these circumstances it may bring reality to the phrase killing with kindness. Oxygen is useful in acute respiratory problems, but for the chronic sufferer it must be used with great caution. Caution will often mean that O_2 would be prescribed by a doctor in low dosage, and the patient monitored closely for respiratory deterioration (Forbes-Faulkner 1998).

Heart diseases can be a cause of increased respiratory rate, including **heart** (or **cardiac**) **failure**. **Left heart failure** (or **left ventricular failure, LVF**) causes blood to accumulate in the pulmonary veins awaiting the opportunity to get into the left side of the heart. This 'traffic jam' of blood gets back to the lungs, where fluid from the plasma can leak into the alveolar spaces causing **pulmonary oedema**. This prevents gas exchange across any alveolar space that is involved in collecting this fluid. This is sometimes referred to as the **backward problem** (see Chapter 2). **Right heart failure (RHF, or congestive cardiac failure, CCF)** can cause increased respiratory rates by reducing the amount of blood being pumped to the lungs, at the same time slowing down circulation in the tissues. The tissues become starved of O_2 and cannot pass their CO_2 quickly to the blood for excretion, and the resulting changes in the Po_2 and Pco_2 affect the respiratory centre. In acidosis, low blood pH (i.e. below the normal of pH 7.4) causes increased respiration in an attempt to remove CO_2 gas from the blood. Carbon dioxide is the acid gas since it combines with water to form carbonic acid, which liberates hydrogen ions (see p. 75).

Increased respiration also occurs as a result of lung collapse (**atelectasis**), which can be due to chest trauma or can occur spontaneously. A **tension pneumothorax** is where air is sucked in through a chest wound and builds up in the pleura, collapsing the lungs; a **pneumothorax** is air in the pleura from a burst **bulla**, or air blister, within the visceral layer. A simple fractured rib can increase respiration rates because the patient cannot take deep breaths owing to the pain and compensates by faster but shallow breathing . Respiratory changes due to the pain of fractured ribs may be inconvenient to the young but could be life threatening to an elderly patient with other respiratory problems, such as chronic bronchitis.

Since blood tends to reach all the alveoli, the efficiency of gas exchange also depends on air reaching all the alveoli as well. This actually varies slightly, with more air than blood occurring in the apex of the lung, and more blood than air occurring in the basal areas. The best blood–air flow match occurs in the central regions, although fine tuning of the air flow to match the blood flow throughout the lungs means that small variations make little difference. However, big differences occur when serious air–blood flow disturbances take place, as in **shunting**. Here, blood passes through big areas of unventilated alveoli, returning from the lungs without any gas exchange. This high P_{CO_2}/low P_{O_2} blood then mixes with blood that has exchanged gases, altering the blood gas tensions of arterial blood (a good example of arterial blood gases being a measure of lung function efficiency). If shunting is severe enough, it will affect oxygenation of the tissues, causing respiratory increases, cyanosis and dyspnoea. Shunting occurs in atelectasis, fluid accumulating in the alveoli, such as in **lobar pneumonia** or pulmonary oedema, or in tension pneumothorax. Lobar pneumonia is a lung infection characterised by exudate (leaked fluid accumulating in the tissues) collecting in the alveoli and preventing air from entering the gas exchange compartment. **Bronchial pneumonia** is similar, where the fluid collects in the bronchus, higher up the respiratory tract. A tidal volume that is too low (i.e. very shallow breathing) is also important as an estimate of respiratory efficiency. Low inhaled volumes will be mostly dead space with little alveolar air. A slow respiratory rate associated with deep breathing can be a feature of some periods of sleep. If slow rates are accompanied by shallow breaths, i.e. low tidal volume, which means low alveolar air volumes, this indicates poor respiratory efficiency. This kind of breathing pattern is very serious, and it is often seen when the patient is close to death. If it happens during sleep, as sometimes is the case, it is known as **sleep apnoea** (apnoea = cessation of breathing), a potential complication that should be investigated (Strohl 1996).

Peak flow

When asked, 'What does a **peak flow** meter measure?' a common answer is that it measures an air volume of some kind. This is not the case, however, as peak flow measures air *speed*, or more exactly, the maximum speed (peak) of air leaving the lungs (flow) during a *forced* expiration. Like a car speed, where a distance is *compared with a time* (miles or kilometres *per hour*), so peak flow compares an air volume *with a time* (litres *per minute*). The adult variation for peak flow is large, owing to differences in sex, age, build, smoking habits, and so on. The average adult peak flow is about 400 litres per minute, with men's values usually slightly higher than women's. Four hundred litres is a large volume, much bigger than any human lungs could contain. In addition, the expiration used to gain this result lasts only a second or two, with only a few litres leaving the lungs. Since the meter is not measuring *all* the 400 litres, the result is an *assumption* that 400 litres *would be* expelled from the lungs if the current maximum speed *had been* maintained for 60 seconds. The value is dependent on healthy **lung compliance**, the lungs' ability to stretch to accommodate incoming air, and on the patency of the air passages. Reduced lung compliance, which limits the lungs' air capacity, or partial airway obstruction (e.g. an asthma attack) will reduce the peak flow significantly. A narrow airway will significantly reduce the speed that air can achieve when leaving the lungs. Peak flow is achieved by blowing as hard and as fast as possible into a peak flow meter, after taking the greatest possible deep breath (inspiratory reserve volume). The full peak flow involves expelling as much of the vital capacity as quickly as possible. The accepted result is the best of three attempts. Severely breathless patients may not be able to perform this test, and it is therefore better used as a predictor of deteriorating respiratory performance before an acute attack.

Cough

Coughing and sneezing are respiratory phenomena with a purpose: that of clearing the airway of obstructions or irritants. The cough reflex centre is in the medulla, in association with the respiratory centre, and initiates coughing from stimuli received from the upper respiratory tract. Choking is an emergency that may occur after the failure of severe coughing to relieve an acute upper respiratory obstruction, such as food. But coughing can also be chronic and persistent, and the nurse should look for a pattern that will shed light on the cause of the cough. Some information needs to be known:

1 Is the cough dry (nothing coughed up) or productive (coughing produces something from the lungs)?

2 Is the cough accompanied by a sore throat or hoarse voice?

A dry cough suggests that a throat irritation is the cause, possibly an **upper respiratory tract infection** (**URTI**) such as the common cold. A sore throat and a hoarse (or lost) voice would further confirm this scenario. A productive cough recovers some substance, usually mucus, from the lungs, suggesting the problem is probably lower in the respiratory system.

Mucous could be substantial, as is often the case with chronic bronchitis, being coughed up every few minutes throughout the day. It may be infected, being mixed with pus, and may appear green. Blood coughed from the lungs (**haemoptysis**) is potentially very serious on two counts: i.e. it is blood lost from circulation potentially causing shock, and it fills the airway preventing inhalation and gas exchange. The result can be death if there is much bleeding and it is not treated quickly. Haemoptysis has various causes: **lung cancer** that has eroded through a main blood vessel; left ventricular failure, where a backflow of blood creates pulmonary congestion; or erosion and enlargement of alveolar lung tissue (**emphysema**) caused by the persistent long-term cough of chronic bronchitis. Emphysema is a permanent complication of smoking that causes chronic dyspnoea. Since smoking is a lung irritant, it is a major cause of several lung and heart disorders, such as cancer, chronic bronchitis, emphysema and coronary thrombosis; knowledge of a patient's history of smoking is important in any lung assessment as smoking could be the reason for many chronic coughs with mucus production.

Respiratory sounds

Respiration is essentially silent, so nurses observing any sounds that occur during breathing should report their findings, with the understanding of what they could represent. **Rales** are crackles or bubbling noises heard mostly on inspiration when air enters parts of the airway that has abnormal fluid present, as in pulmonary oedema due to heart failure or pneumonia. They are unaffected by coughing. **Rhonchi** are wheezes heard mostly on expiration and often clear after coughing. High-pitched rhonchi (**sibilant rhonchi**) come from the small branches of the respiratory passages and are heard, for example, in patients suffering from asthma. Lower-pitched rhonchi (**sonorous rhonchi**) are from the larger bronchi and occur in **bronchitis**. These sounds can be identified using auscultation, i.e. listening to the chest through a stethoscope, but severe forms of the sound may be heard while in close proximity to the patient without any listening aids. Such observations should be reported urgently to the doctor since intervention may be necessary to improve the patient's breathing. **Stridor** is one such urgent problem; it is a loud, harsh, high-pitched and vibrating sound, sometimes called crowing, during mostly inspiration, and caused by partial obstruction of the larynx (**laryngeal stridor**) or trachea. Sometimes this can happen in newborn babies and is known as **congenital laryngeal stridor**. The cause in the newborn is a congenital defect of the upper opening of the larynx, but the sound usually disappears by around 1 year of age. Stridor can be heard in **croup**, an acute upper-respiratory (larynx and trachea) infection, which is often viral in origin, and affects mostly children. It is accompanied by dyspnoea and distress, and sometimes sternal and ribcage retraction, when the chest wall is pulled back during inspiration. If inadequate air reaches the lungs, cyanosis may occur.

Cyanosis

Cyanosis is generally regarded as a grey, blue or mauve discoloration of the skin, depending on the degree of severity (Carpenter 1993). It is caused by a lack of oxygen in the tissues (**tissue hypoxia**), but the skin colour change is due to an accumulation of **reduced haemoglobin** in the tissues. Reduced haemoglobin is haemoglobin without oxygen that takes on a hydrogen ion (H^+) in order to buffer these ions and prevent pH changes in the circulation (see blood gas transport p. 75 and Chapter 1). Excess reduced haemoglobin occurs as a result of inadequate oxygenation, when there is an excess of vacant haemoglobin capable of binding hydrogen ions. In general, if the colour change is observed in the periphery (i.e. the hands and feet) this is due to normal adequate arterial blood oxygenation, but the tissues are extracting excess oxygen from this blood, leaving larger than normal quantities of reduced haemoglobin in the venules. These tiny veins contribute to the visible colour of the skin. Restriction of blood supply to a part or whole of a limb may cause a degree of peripheral cyanosis in that affected limb. If the cyanosis is observed more centrally (i.e. the trunk or face) it is due to the lack of oxygenation of arterial blood by the lungs. The greater the volume of reduced haemoglobin, the more severe is the colour change from grey to deep purple. Central cyanosis can be treated with oxygen, which will occupy larger quantities of haemoglobin and therefore lower the level of reduced haemoglobin in the tissues.

Oxygen blood saturation (pulse oximetry)

Each haemoglobin molecule in the blood can bind and carry four oxygen molecules to the tissues, and as such haemoglobin would be 100% saturated. A haemoglobin molecule with only three oxygen molecules is 75% saturated, with two oxygen molecules it is 50% saturated, and so on. A mixture of haemoglobin molecules, some at 100%, some at 75%, some at 50%, and so on, results in a saturation value for *whole* blood at figures between those stated, e.g. 95% saturated. The amount of oxygen carried on haemoglobin should normally be very close to 100% (i.e. fully saturated). This can be monitored easily by attaching the patient's finger to a clip-on sensor that gives an instant readout of both the pulse and oxygen saturation level: the pulse oximeter. Low levels of oxygen saturation, e.g. less than 97%, indicate a problem in the lungs that is preventing full oxygenation of the blood. Such problems include many of the lung conditions discussed here, such as chronic bronchitis and pneumonia. The importance of this on-the-spot method of noting the oxygen saturation when compared with repeated arterial blood sampling and the delay while awaiting the results becomes obvious. Rapid changes in oxygen saturation can be detected quickly and corrective treatment can be carried out at once. Oxygen saturation of blood is affected by the blood gas tension of oxygen (Po_2), and a correlation of oxygen saturations over a range of Po_2 is shown by the oxygen saturation curve (Figure 4.7). The difference between the two is that saturation involves the *volume* of oxygen carried, whereas the gas tension is the *pressure* it exerts. Naturally, the greater the volume carried, the greater is the pressure exerted. The curve shows a high saturation (98.5%) in the lungs giving a Po_2 of 100 mmHg, and a lower saturation (75%) in the tissues giving a lower Po_2 of 40 mmHg (see blood gas tensions p. 79). This represents an off-loading of oxygen in the tissues that desaturates haemoglobin by about 23%, and a corresponding on-loading of oxygen in the lungs. Shifts in this curve occur as a result of various changes in physical parameters, as indicated in Figure 4.7, and understanding of the curve and its variations will aid in interpreting abnormalities of the pulse oximetry.

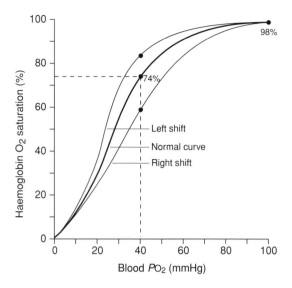

FIGURE 4.7 The oxygen saturation curve. The percentage of oxygen saturation of haemoglobin is plotted against the oxygen blood gas tension (PO_2). The normal curve (centre) shows an off-loading of oxygen to the tissues from 98% to 74% saturated (PO_2 of tissues being approximately 40 mmHg) and a loading of oxygen to the haemoglobin from 74% to 98% saturation in the lungs (PO_2 of the lungs being approximately 100 mmHg). Shifts of the curve to the left or right can happen (see text).

Childhood breathing

Normal respiration rates vary in childhood according to age. At birth, the rate is from 30 to 80, in early childhood it is from 20 to 40 and in late childhood from 15 to 25. All the infant lung volumes are much smaller than the adult, the tidal volume being about 15 ml, with a corresponding smaller dead space. Diaphragmatic breathing is dominant over chest wall movements during the early years of life, and as a result the nurse may find it easier to count abdominal movements rather than chest wall movements. Respiratory effort forms part of the **Apgar score** carried out at birth to assess the infant's condition, (i.e. 0 = absent breathing, 1 = gasping or irregular breathing, 2 = crying or rhythmic breathing) (Figure 4.8) (Letko 1996). Breathing responses to illness, exercise and emotion are greater in children than in adults. Premature infants may suffer respiratory problems because their lung development is incomplete. Probably the commonest respiratory symptom in children is coughing, which is usually caused by a throat irritation or a mild **upper respiratory tract infection (URTI)**, such as the common cold. Just occasionally it may be more serious, e.g. pneumonia (Kambarami *et al.* 1996).

Assessment	Score		
	0	1	2
Heart rate	Absent	Slow (<100/min)	Over 100/min
Respiratory effort	Absent	Slow or irregular	Good crying
Muscle tone	Limp	Some flexion of extremities	Action motion
Response to stimulation	None	Poor, with grimace	Good crying
Colour	Blue or pale	Body pink extremities blue	Completely pink

Score 0–3 = severe distress of infant
Score 4–7 = moderate distress of infant
Score 8–10 = no difficulty of infant to adjust to extrauterine life

FIGURE 4.8 The Apgar score.

The child who is born before full term is *premature*, and as a result may suffer severe respiratory problems. **Hyaline membrane disease (HMD)** is due to a lack of **surfactant** on the alveolar wall. Lungs must switch from being fluid filled to air filled at birth, and surfactant produced in the lungs lowers the resistance of the alveolar wall to stretching (i.e. it lowers the **surface tension**). A lack of surfactant results in lungs that will not expand properly and therefore will not admit air. It results in **respiratory distress syndrome (RDS)**, a complication seen in very preterm babies, i.e. those with immature lungs, but the condition is rare after 37 weeks' gestation. RDS involves respiratory rates over 100 breaths per minute, expiratory **grunting** sounds (due to expiration against a partially closed **glottis**, the narrowest part of the airway inside the larynx) and chest wall retraction. In severe cases the baby is cyanosed with gasping respirations and even apnoea and will need resuscitation, oxygen and assisted breathing, possibly ventilation. Hypoxia must be prevented because it can cause brain damage and less surfactant production; a high oxygen level is also dangerous since it can cause blindness by damaging the retina. Oxygen supplementation should be medically prescribed and strictly monitored.

Young children are more prone than adults to lung infections, mostly because they have an immature immune system which is exposed to a world of infectious agents (**antigens**) that are new to them. Some conditions, like **cystic fibrosis**, make this problem worse. Cystic fibrosis is a genetic congenital disorder of exocrine gland secretion that affects mostly the mucus of the lungs and digestive system. Mucous becomes thick and sticky, with repeated infections, not only causing malabsorption and malnutrition but also chronic respiratory obstruction with breathing difficulty. Children born with the condition previously had a limited life expectancy, but now they are surviving into adulthood as a result of the advances that have been made in care and treatment.

Key points

- We need oxygen (O_2) from the air, but the primary driving force of breathing is carbon dioxide (CO_2).
- In acidosis, blood below pH 7.4 causes increased respiration in an attempt to remove carbon dioxide, an acid gas, from the circulation.
- Movement of gases across the alveoli uses gas concentration gradients.
- The lungs are held tightly against the chest wall by a negative pressure, or vacuum, existing between the visceral and parietal layers of the pleura.
- The volume of air taken in with each breath is the tidal volume, about 500 ml in adults, subdivided into the alveolar air, which will exchange gas, about 350 ml, and the dead space, which will not exchange gas, about 150 ml.
- Respiration depends on the respiratory centre, which is shared between the medulla and the pons, in the brain stem.
- The average respiratory rate in an adult is about 15–18 times per minute, but the rate can rise to > 30 times per minute during exercise or when there is a respiratory or a cardiac disorder. Breathing consists of an inspiration, an expiration and a brief pause.
- Oxygen and carbon dioxide in the blood create a gas pressure, the blood gas tensions. The P_{O_2} of arterial blood is 13.3 kPa, or 100 mmHg; the P_{CO_2} is 5.3 kPa, or 40 mmHg. Venous blood P_{O_2} = 5.3 kPa or 40 mmHg; P_{CO_2} = 6.1 kPa or 46 mmHg.
- Pneumothorax is air in the pleural space.
- Left heart failure (LVF) causes blood to back up into the pulmonary veins, and fluid from the plasma leaks into the alveoli causing pulmonary oedema and dyspnoea.
- Shunting involves blood passing through areas of unventilated alveoli, returning from the lungs without any gas exchange.

- Cyanosis is a grey to mauve discoloration of the skin caused by a lack of oxygen resulting in an accumulation in the tissues of reduced haemoglobin (i.e. haemoglobin that has a hydrogen ion attached).
- Stridor is a loud, harsh high-pitched sound during inspiration caused by partial obstruction of the larynx (laryngeal stridor) or trachea.
- Peak flow measures the maximum speed of air leaving the lungs during a forced expiration.
- Respiration is silent. Nurses observing abnormal breath sounds should report their findings, with the understanding of what they represent.
- Respiratory distress syndrome (RDS) is sometimes seen in very preterm babies. It involves respiratory rates over 100 per minute, expiratory grunting and chest wall retraction. In severe cases cyanosis with gasping respirations and even apnoea occur.
- Smoking is a lung irritant and a major cause of lung cancer, chronic bronchitis, emphysema and heart diseases. Knowledge of a patient's smoking history is important in any lung assessment.

References

Carpenter K. D. (1993) A comprehensive review of cyanosis. *Critical Care Nurse*, 13(4): 66–72.

Forbes-Faulkner L. (1998) Oxygen Therapy: challenges for nurses. *Kai-Tiaki: Nursing New Zealand*, 4(3): 17–19.

Grey A. (1995) Breathless...dyspnoea. *Nursing Times*, July 5th; 91(27): 46–47.

Hickey J. V. (1997) *The Clinical Practice of Neurological and Neurosurgical Nursing*, 4th edn. J. B. Lippincott Company, Philadelphia.

Kambarami R. A., Rusakaniko S. and Mahomva L. A. (1996) Ability of caregivers to recognise signs of pneumonia in coughing children aged below five years. *Central African Journal of Medicine*, 42(10): 291–294.

Letko M. D. (1996) Understanding the Apgar score. *Journal of Obstetric, Gynecologic and Neonatal Nursing*, 25(4): 299–303.

Owen A. 1998 Respiratory Assessment revisited. *Nursing*, 28(4): 48–49.

Strohl K. P. 1996 The biology of sleep apnea. *Science and Medicine*, Sept/Oct: 32–41.

Chapter 5

Elimination (I): urinary observations

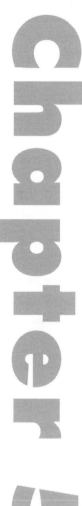

- Introduction
- Urine formation
- Urinary observations
- Urinary volume
- Colour, smell and deposits
- Specific gravity
- Urinalysis
- When to test urine

Introduction

The eliminatory systems are the body's principal excretory pathways for many surplus and toxic substances produced from a wide variety of tissues. Their functions are crucial in the maintenance of the body's tissue and blood contents at permanently optimum levels essential for life. It is natural that the body should excrete products generated not only in health but as a result of pathology, and the nurse must be familiar with the normal and abnormal states of the eliminated product. Urine, for example, a seemingly waste material, offers a unique insight into the physiological workings of many body systems. Accurate observations of urine can reveal much about the individual at that time, both the factors affecting the system and the underlying metabolism.

Urine formation

The formation of urine is the role of the **nephron** (Figure 5.1), of which there are about one million in each of the two kidneys. Urine production takes place in three distinct steps.

Step 1 is **filtration under pressure** in the **glomerulus**, which is surrounded by the **glomerular (Bowman's) capsule** (Figure 5.2). Blood plasma passing through the glomerular arterioles is subject to **hydrostatic pressure** (i.e. blood pressure as it occurs in the glomerular arterioles) causing filtration by forcing water and other substances through the **glomerular membrane**. The resulting filtrate is collected in the capsule at a rate known as the **glomerular filtration rate (GFR)**, which is about 120 ml per minute, measured as a total of all two million nephrons. Water and other small molecules may pass through the membrane, including sodium and glucose, but large molecules, such as most proteins and blood cells, cannot pass through and remain in the blood.

Step 2 is the re-absorption of required substances, including much of the water, back into the circulation from the **proximal convoluted tubule** (Figure 5.3). Water returns to the blood at a rate of about 105 ml per minute, measured as a total of all two million nephrons. Other substances returned include sodium and all of the glucose. The remaining filtrate passes into the **loop of Henle**, which has the effect of causing an osmotic gradient across the renal cortex that becomes important to water re-absorption from the straight collecting ducts (Figure 5.4). Filtrate then passes into the **distal convoluted tubule**, where further re-absorption of substances takes place, some of which

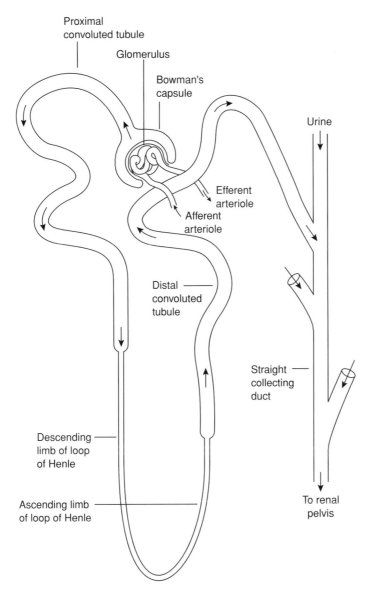

FIGURE 5.1 The renal nephron. The glomerulus, inside the Bowman's capsule, is formed from a tuft of arterioles; the blood enters via the afferent arteriole and leaves via the efferent arteriole. Filtrate flows along the proximal convoluted tubule to the loop of Henle, passing down the descending limb and up the ascending limb. The distal convoluted tubule conveys filtrate to the straight collecting duct, where, as urine, it flows to the renal pelvis and to the bladder.

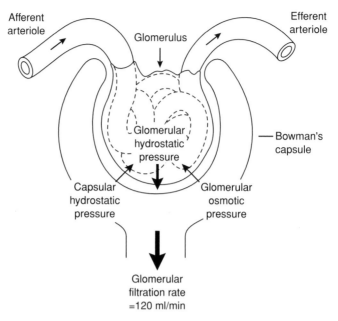

Figure 5.2 The glomerulus and Bowman's capsule. The glomerulus is covered by a filtration membrane. Water is pushed out of the blood and into the Bowman's capsule by the glomerular hydrostatic pressure (GHP). Two other forces are returning water to the blood. The capsular hydrostatic pressure is the pressure of the fluid within the capsule, and the glomerular osmotic pressure is the force exerted by the proteins within the blood to attract water back. The GHP is greater than the sum of the other two, creating a glomerular filtration rate of approximately 120 ml/min, measured as a sum total for all two million nephrons (one million per kidney).

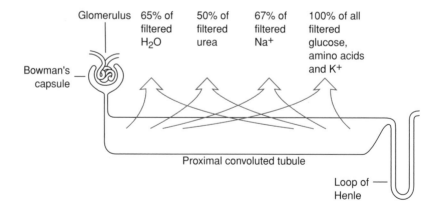

Figure 5.3 The proximal convoluted tubule, between the Bowman's capsule and the loop of Henle re-absorbs water, urea, sodium and other substances. The percentage shown is that of the amount filtered by the glomerulus.

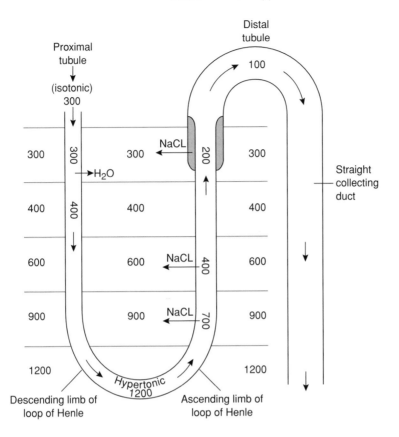

All figures in mosmol/l
(milliosmoles per litre)

FIGURE 5.4 The loop of Henle passes through a sodium concentration gradient outside the loop caused by blood capillaries called the vasa recta, which follow the loop closely (not shown). The concentration gradient is shown from 300 to 1200 mosmol/l. Water can pass out of the descending limb but not the ascending limb, and sodium is unable to pass out of the descending limb but is actively transported out of the ascending limb. The filtrate passing down the descending limb is isotonic to begin with but becomes more concentrated in sodium (i.e. hypertonic) as water is lost. As the filtrate returns up the ascending limb sodium is lost and it becomes less concentrated. The resultant dilution of the filtrate in the distal convoluted tubule (100 mosmol/l) allows the kidney to excrete urine more dilute than body fluids (hypotonic) when necessary. The gradient along the straight collecting duct allows the kidney to reclaim water (under antidiuretcic hormone control) and therefore excrete urine more concentrated than body fluids (hypertonic) when necessary (see Figures 5.5, 5.6 and 5.7).

is under hormonal control. The re-absorption of water is controlled by **antidiuretic hormone (ADH)** and that of sodium by **aldosterone** (Figure 5.5). ADH is also active along the straight collecting ducts controlling water re-absorption in response to the osmotic gradient mentioned earlier.

Step 3 involves the addition of certain substances, notably hydrogen ions (H^+) (see p. 75), ammonia (NH_3) (see p. 8) and potassium ions (K^+) into the filtrate from the blood by means of **tubular secretion**, which takes place in the **straight collecting ducts**. The resultant filtrate is now urine, which then passes to the renal pelvis and into the bladder for elimination.

Urinary observations

Nurses in most clinical areas will observe the volume, colour, smell, deposits and specific gravity of urine and perform chemical tests for glucose, pH, protein, blood, bilirubin, urobilinogen, ketones, nitrite and leucocytes. Collecting urinary specimens and the use of reagent testing strips are described by Walsh (1989), Lloyd (1993) and Cook (1995). The correct technique cannot be overemphasised, since the

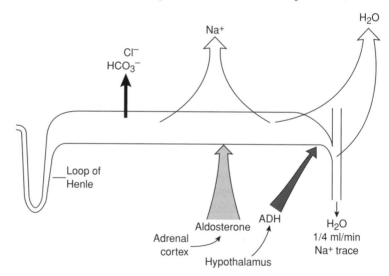

Figure 5.5 The distal convoluted tubule. After the loop of Henle the distal tubule absorbs chlorine (Cl^-) and bicarbonate (HCO_3^-). Sodium (Na^+) is re-absorbed under aldosterone control from the adrenal cortex, and water (H_2O) is re-absorbed under the control of antidiuretic hormone (ADH) from the hypothalamus. The amount of water returned to the blood allows an average of one-quarter of a millilitre per hour as urine production.

reagent test strips are calibrated to perform accurately within precise limits, and they will give false results if used wrongly. These limits include using the strips before the expiry dates, storage in a dry environment and reading the results at the specified time limit (usually 60 seconds). Holding the strip the correct way round when comparing the reactive pads with the colour chart is another vital point so often overlooked by those who are new to the procedure. Testing freshly voided urine is another critical point, since urine constituents change with time when left standing, especially when exposed to the air. Again, false results occur when testing old urine. The accuracy of the reagent strips is discussed by Cook (1996) and Wells (1997).

Urinary volume

Between them the two kidneys produce urine at the average rate of 1 ml per minute given an average oral intake of fluids. Variations in oral intake will change this output volume by adjusting the levels of ADH in the blood. ADH is produced by the hypothalamus of the brain and moves to the posterior pituitary gland. From here it is released into the circulation and acts on the straight collecting ducts leading from the nephrons. The role of ADH is to facilitate the return of water from the urinary filtrate to the blood, thus controlling the concentration of urine, and it is therefore a major influence on fluid balance in the body. It works by binding to ADH receptors on the surface of cells lining the straight collecting duct, cells which also have a surface close to the local blood circulation. Binding of ADH activates intracellular systems that open channels specific to water on the cell surfaces facing the filtrate. Water passes down these channels into the cell, driven by the osmotic gradient set up by the loop of Henle. From there, water passes back into the blood. After the GFR of 120 ml per minute and the re-absorption of water from the proximal convoluted tubule, the remaining filtrate has a water volume of about 15 ml per minute. Average ADH levels, as found in those who are drinking normal amounts daily, return about 14 ml per minute to the blood, leaving an average of 1 ml per minute as urine. But let us consider the extremes of ADH activity as seen in those persons with very different oral intakes of fluid. Mr Wet is in the pub drinking multiple pints in quick succession (Figure 5.6). His high oral intake of fluid (mostly water) sends stimuli to the hypothalamus to reduce ADH production and release, and it thus lowers the amount that is active on the kidneys. A minimum of

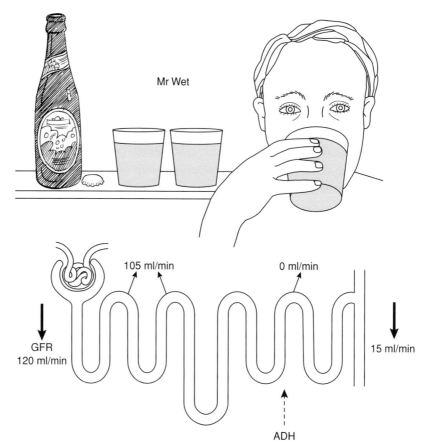

FIGURE 5.6 Mr Wet physiology. If a large volume of fluid is drunk, the kidney can compensate by excreting more urine. The figures are totals for the two million nephrons (one million per kidney). The glomerular filtration rate (GFR) is approximately 120 ml/min, and the first tubule re-absorption rate is approximately 105 ml/min. The variations begin in the distal tubule because of very low levels of antidiuretic hormone (ADH). Signals to the brain have caused a shutdown of ADH production and release. As little or none of the water in the distal tubule can be returned to the blood, giving a urine output of 15 ml/min, the renal maximum.

ADH release can be achieved if the oral intake is high enough. Less water is returned from the collecting duct as a result, i.e. little or no post-loop re-absorption occurs, and the urine output increases to a maximum of 15 ml per minute, the **renal maximum** (a **polyuria**, or **diuresis**). Outputs higher than this suggest that the kidneys have lost control of fluid balance, a feature of **chronic renal failure**. Failure here means failure to control fluid balance. As Mr Wet's drink contains alcohol, this will have a further dehydrating effect during the following few hours by suppressing ADH production. Dehydration is said to be one of the causes of the hangover. Meanwhile, poor Mr Dry is crawling through the desert, with no oral fluids, and he is losing a great deal of water through his skin by sweating in the hot sun. The fizzy drinks machines he sees are, unfortunately for him, all mirages. His low oral intake of fluid causes stimuli to pass to the hypothalamus causing an increase in the production and release of ADH, therefore boosting his ADH activity on the kidneys (Figure 5.7). Up to 14.75 ml per minute

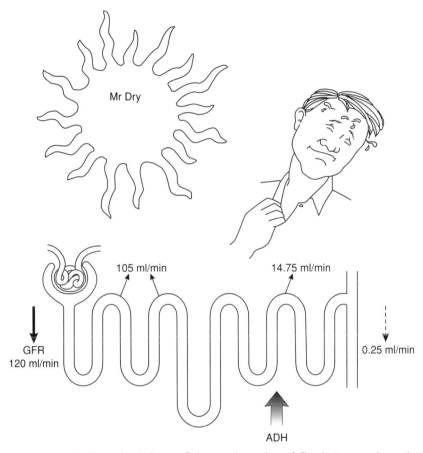

FIGURE 5.7 Mr Dry physiology. If the oral intake of fluids is very low, the kidney can compensate to prevent unnecessary water loss. The figures shown are totals for the two million nephrons (one million per kidney). The glomerular filtration rate (GFR) is approximately 120 ml/minute; the re-absorption rate from the first tubule is about 105 ml/min. The difference begins in the second tubule when large amounts of antidiuretic hormone (ADH) are active, returning up to 14.75 ml/min water to the blood and creating a urine output of only one-quarter of a millilitre per minute, the renal minimum.

of the post-loop 15 ml per minute filtrate can be returned leaving a urine output of about 0.25 ml per minute, the **renal minimum** (an **oliguria**). Zero output (**anuria**) is not possible in normal renal physiology as this would cause retention of wastes, especially urea, a feature of **acute renal failure**. Here, the word failure means failure to produce urine, otherwise known as renal shutdown.

Nurses can observe urine volume outputs in relation to total fluid balance in those patients at most risk of imbalance, i.e. those who are nil by mouth or are not drinking well; those on intravenous infusion; those with excessive fluid losses from sweating, overbreathing, bleeding or drains; and those with renal disease or children with diarrhoea and vomiting. Outputs falling below 1 ml per minute (60 ml per hour) should be monitored closely and medical advice sought if the output reaches 30 ml or less per hour. High outputs should return to normal as fluid balance is restored, but outputs remaining consistently high, or exceeding 15 ml per minute (900 ml per hour), particularly if the input is not high, should be referred for medical advice. One cause of polyuria is **diabetes**, the word means a disease characterised by a large urine output. Since more than one disorder causes a polyuria, at least two distinct diabetic diseases are recognised. **Diabetes insipidus** is a polyuria caused by a lack of ADH owing to failure of the hypothalamus or pituitary. The urine tests negative for glucose (thus *insipidus*, i.e. insipid = not sweet) compared with the sweet urine of **diabetes mellitus** (melli = honey), where glucose in the urine (**glycosuria**) is a major feature and the cause of the polyuria. Glucose-laden filtrate within the nephron tubule exerts an osmotic force that retains the water present in the filtrate and attracts more water out of the blood, all of which escapes as urine. The resultant state of dehydration causes thirst, a reversal of the normal condition, when the oral fluid input drives the renal output (Figure 5.8).

Diuretic drugs are those that induce a diuresis for medical purposes, i.e. to treat **hypertension** or **cardiac failure** that is causing **oedema**. Several groups of drugs achieve a large urine output, and nurses should be aware that such an output is expected from this treatment and warn the patients accordingly. The **thiazides** (e.g. **bendroflumethiazide** and **hydrochlorothiazide**) prevent the re-absorption of sodium from the distal parts of the tubule. The sodium remains in the filtrate and is lost in the urine. Water follows sodium, so a sodium loss creates a diuresis. **Loop diuretics** (e.g. **frusemide** and **bumetanide**) work by preventing re-absorption of sodium at the loop of Henle. They are the most potent

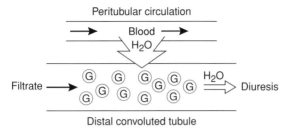

Peritubular circulation

Distal convoluted tubule

FIGURE 5.8 Mechanism of the large urine loss (diuresis) in uncontrolled diabetes. Glucose is not normally present in the distal convoluted tubule, so if glucose molecules (G) do get through to this part of the nephron they cause a return of water (H_2O) from the peritubular blood circulation to the filtrate. This osmotic increase in filtrate water causes the large urine loss (diuresis) that is seen in uncontrolled diabetes.

diuretics, producing the largest urine outputs but with the greatest potential for causing unwanted reactions. They may promote the loss of potassium as well, and this can be a complication. The **potassium-sparing** diuretics (e.g. **amiloride** and **spironolactone**) conserve potassium while causing mild diuresis as a result of sodium loss. In addition, spironolactone is an aldosterone **antagonist**, i.e. it reduces the activity of aldosterone and this promotes further sodium and water loss.

Colour, smell and deposits

The normal colour of urine is a clear pale yellow with no clouding or deposits. Urine density affects the colour: the more dilute the urine is with water the weaker the colour. Concentrated urine becomes darker, depending on how much pigment is present. This is normal, but the colour can also change when unusual substances are present (see Plate 1, facing p. 114). **Bilirubin** will stain the urine a strong yellow colour, and when seen in bulk in concentrated urine it can appear to be black. Bilirubin is the end product of the breakdown of haemoglobin from erythrocytes (red blood cells) in circulation (see bilirubin and urobilinogen p. 107). Whole blood will change the colour according to the amount present and how long it has been mixed with urine. Small amounts of blood added to the urine during formation, i.e. well mixed with urine in the kidney, may give a grey smoky appearance, whereas larger amounts added lower down the renal tract will look like true blood, giving red urine (**haematuria**, see p. 106). Red urine may also be a feature of excessive beetroot consumption in the diet, and

101

some drugs may affect the colour, e.g. anthraquinones in laxatives such as senna may turn urine yellow, brown or orange. Ford (1992) gives a comprehensive list of urine colours and the causes, including many drugs, the result of considerable research in this area.

Both **urea** and **ammonia** are nitrogenous (i.e. contain nitrogen) wastes of protein metabolism, normally produced by the liver from excess protein. Ammonia is more toxic that urea and gives a more powerful smell. The ammonia smell associated with some urine specimens is due to infective organisms in the urinary tract (a **urinary tract infection**, or **UTI**) that split the urea molecules present in urine into ammonia. Urine can smell of acetone if left to stand for some hours, the result of collecting organisms from the environment and a good reason for testing only fresh samples. **Ketones** are waste products of fat (lipid) metabolism, the main ketone being **acetone**, which gives the urine a pear drop or nail-polish remover smell. This is usually present in association with glycosuria in diabetes mellitus (see p. 107).

Deposits are another indication of a potential problem with urine. Cloudy urine in UTIs is caused by the presence of inflammatory cells (leucocytes), bacteria (both live and dead), pus, mucus and cellular debris. Alternatively, excessive calcium excretion can give a cloudy effect and leave a chalky deposit on standing. This may be due to excessive calcium in the diet or to any of the decalcifying bone diseases, such as **osteoporosis**. Here, too much calcium leaves the bone and passes to the kidneys via the blood and is excreted in the urine; patients are said to be *urinating their skeleton*. Excessive calcium lost in urine also increases that person's risk of forming renal stones. Phosphates and **urates** (salts of **uric acid**) can produce cloudy effects in urine. Uric acid is the excretory product from the breakdown of nucleic acids such as **deoxyribonucleic acid (DNA)** and **ribonucleic acid (RNA)**. **Casts** can also leave a visible deposit when urine is left to stand. Casts are made from a matrix of a mucoprotein produced by the distal tubular epithelium that fills and takes the shape of the tubule lumen. Cells get incorporated into this matrix, which can then be washed out by the urine. When excreted, these casts indicate a potentially high protein content and a low urinary pH. When cloudy urine is observed, a sample should be collected for laboratory analysis to determine the exact component and its cause.

Specific gravity

The **density** of urine identifies how much **solute** there is present. Solutes are chemical substances that are dissolved in the water component, such as sodium chloride (found in trace quantities in urine). Specific gravity is the measure of a urine's density compared with the density of pure water (see Plate 2, facing p. 114). By using water as a baseline density, the specific gravity of urine states just how much more dense than water a certain urine sample is. Since the fluid component of urine is water, the specific gravity measures the volume of dissolved solutes in that water. The baseline density of water is 1000 (or 1.000, labelled 0 on some hydrometers), and a particular urine sample will measure greater than this, e.g. 1010, (or 1.010) if the hydrometer reads 10. The normal range of specific gravity for urine is 1002 (or 1.002) for dilute urine, to 1035 (or 1.035) for concentrated urine (p. 97). The **hydrometer** (or **urinometer**) floats in the urine sample with the large bulb downwards, and measurement is made from where the urine surface crosses the stem scale (see Plate 3, facing p. 115). How high (in dense urine) or how low (in dilute urine) the urinometer floats is an indication of how much the urine is pushing back against the weight of the instrument, and this is the effect of the solute content. Think of the difference between a body floating in the swimming pool (low solute density) and floating in the Dead Sea (high solute density).

The specific gravity is affected by both the water concentration and the solute concentration in the urine sample. The water concentration varies as described (see p. 97). Solutes vary in concentration, depending on several factors because many different solutes are involved. **Sodium (Na$^+$)** is naturally excreted from the kidneys in amounts according to blood levels of sodium and its controlling hormone, **aldosterone**. A high oral intake of sodium chloride (NaCl) increases the blood level, which promotes removal of more sodium by glomerular filtration. The majority of the filtered sodium will return to the blood from the proximal convoluted tubule; most of the remainder will be re-absorbed from the distal convoluted tubule under aldosterone control. Aldosterone comes from the adrenal cortex, and is released according to blood sodium levels: higher levels reduce aldosterone release; lower levels increase its release. Aldosterone acts to facilitate sodium re-absorption back into the blood. In high blood sodium levels (**hypernatraemia**) less aldosterone allows more sodium to escape in the urine and reduce the blood level. In low blood sodium levels (**hyponatraemia**) the higher aldosterone release allows more sodium to return to the blood and thereby increase the blood level. Aldosterone release is also facilitated by the **renin–angiotensin–aldosterone** cycle, whereby the kidney emergency hormone renin is produced under low blood pressure or low blood sodium conditions. Renin activates the blood protein angiotensin (a vasoconstrictive agent that raises blood pressure), which in turn also stimulates aldosterone release to conserve sodium. Sodium is filtered and re-absorbed under aldosterone control very much like water and ADH (Table 5.1).

Calcium (**Ca²⁺**), **phosphates** and other solutes are eliminated in the filtrate and contribute to the specific gravity. However, some solutes, such as potassium, are also excreted using a different process. **Potassium (K⁺)** is largely added to urine by tubular secretion using a cellular mechanism that also transports hydrogen (H⁺) (Figure 5.9). This occurs at the straight collecting duct, eliminating the exact amount of these substances required to maintain normal blood levels.

Urinalysis

Eight different chemical tests have been developed to measure the amounts of important solutes in urine that may indicate disease. These are impregnated into pads and mounted on plastic strips in a convenient manner for urine testing (see Plate 4, facing p. 115).

Glucose in urine

Glucose is filtered via the glomerulus and absorbed back into the blood from the proximal convoluted tubule. Under normal circumstances this return to circulation is total, leaving no glucose in the filtrate or urine. The process of absorption involves glucose transport molecules within the cells that line the tubule, and these molecules move glucose from the filtrate back into the blood. A set amount of transport molecules

TABLE 5.1 Water and sodium in urine

Substance	Glomerular filtered	Proximal tubule	Hormone	Distal tubule	Amount in urine
Water	Yes	Most is re-absorbed	ADH	Average 14 ml/min	Average 1 ml/min
Sodium	Yes	Most is re-absorbed	Aldosterone	Most is re-absorbed	Trace

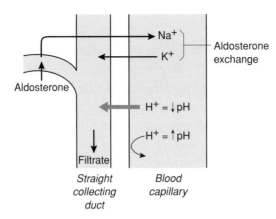

Figure 5.9 Mechanism of aldosterone action. The return of sodium (Na^+) to the blood by aldosterone in the distal convoluted tubule is accompanied by the return of potassium (K^+) to the filtrate (aldosterone exchange). Thus aldosterone influences the potassium balance. In addition, hydrogen ions (H^+) can be returned to the filtrate from the straight collecting duct or retained in the blood, according to the need to maintain the blood pH balance at pH 7.4. Under low pH conditions (e.g. acidosis) hydrogen ions are excreted, and under high pH conditions (alkalosis) hydrogen ions are retained.

means that glucose movement is finite, but this is adequate for the average volume of glucose found in the filtrate under normal conditions. It is possible, sometimes, for glomerular filtration to exceed this **renal threshold** for glucose, and the surplus glucose remaining in the filtrate passes through the remaining nephron and into the urine. This will happen mostly when excess glucose occurs in the blood (**hyperglycaemia**), as in diabetes mellitus. More appears in the filtrate than the transport mechanisms can return to circulation and the renal threshold is exceeded. Glycosuria can also occur during pregnancy, but it is usually of no significance, or in individuals with naturally fewer transport molecules but who do not have diabetes. Glucose is, of course, sweet, and glycosuria makes urine sweet, a fact that was all too obvious to doctors and nurses before the days of chemical tests. They had to test urine by tasting it. Now, health and safety regulations would not allow this, and sophisticated tests such as those described here have, for many years, made this method of testing unnecessary. Modern chemical tests provide a more reliable and accurate alternative. However, keen observation still remains important, like the case of the psychiatric charge nurse who noticed that one patient's urine, when accidentally dripped on the floor, attracted ants. Further investigation revealed that the patient had glycosuria and diabetes.

Protein in urine

Protein does not normally appear in the urine. Blood proteins include **albumin**, which occurs in larger quantities than all the others, and **globulin**, **fibrinogen** and **prothrombin** (the last two are also clotting factors). Protein molecules are, at 7–9 nm, too large to pass through the glomerular membrane pores (about 3 nm). Albumin could pass through the pores but is mostly repelled back into the circulation by the strong negative charges associated with the glycoproteins of the glomerular membrane. What few proteins do appear in the filtrate can be reclaimed by **pinocytosis** (a process similar to phagocytosis) of the urinary cells. Protein in the urine (**proteinuria**, or more specifically **albuminuria**) can be caused by damage to the glomerular membrane, resulting in a larger pore size, such as in glomerular infections (glomerulonephritis), and nephrotoxic agents. Systemic hypertension raises the intraglomerular blood pressure and forces more protein into the filtrate. **Nephrotic syndrome** is a condition recognised by a persistent protein loss in the urine (3.5 g or more of protein lost per day) and can result in a reduced blood protein level with the consequence of tissue oedema.

Blood in the urine

Blood in the urine (**haematuria**) may be normal in some circumstances (e.g. blood contamination of urine during menstruation), or may be expected (e.g. immediately after bladder or prostate surgery) but is often a manifestation of a pathology that requires investigation. Blood in the urine can occur as a result of trauma to any part of the renal system or be caused by the effects of renal stones damaging the urinary wall. Blood can also occur as a result of infections or new growths within the bladder, kidney or prostate gland. The test pad for blood on clinical sticks is sensitive to haemoglobin, ensuring a positive result even when red blood cells have been broken down. Haematuria is often a post-operative feature of bladder, prostate or renal surgery, and it appears as bright red urine (frank blood), diminishing in intensity over several post-operative days until the urine appears normal and blood can only be detected by testing. Eventually, uncomplicated recovery, aided by good fluid input, results in a blood-free urinalysis.

Ketones in urine

Ketones are the end product of excess **adipose** (fat) breakdown in the body. Adipose stores fats in the form of **triglyceride,** which has three fatty acids attached to a glycerol molecule (see Figure 1.4). Normally, fatty acids are repackaged for return to the circulation by the liver. In diabetes mellitus, when a lack of insulin prevents cells from using glucose as an energy source, or in starvation, when glucose is in short supply, adipose is broken down (**lipolysis**) to release more of the fatty acids. Fatty acids can be used as an emergency energy supply by entering the tricarboxylic acid (Krebs) cycle (see Figure 1.1), and in the presence of oxygen they are used to create energy in the form of **adenosine triphosphate (ATP)** (see Chapter 1). Massive release of fatty acids into the circulation results in the liver converting the excess (that which cannot be metabolised to energy), through an anaerobic route, into any of the three human ketones, mostly **acetone**, but also **acetoacetic acid** and **beta-hydroxybutyric acid**. Acetone, being the largest amount produced, is excreted via both the kidneys and the lungs, giving a sweet pear drop smell to the urine and breath, as noted in diabetes mellitus (see Chapter 1).

Bilirubin in the urine

Bilirubin and urobilinogen are products of haemoglobin breakdown when it is released from old destroyed red blood cells (Figure 5.10). **Erythrocytes** (red blood cells) degrade and release haemoglobin after about 120 days in circulation. Haemoglobin is first split into a haem and a globin portion. Globin, a protein, can be reduced to amino acids, and the iron is removed from the haem for storage in the liver. What is left of the haem component is **biliverdin**, which is further converted to bilirubin, which is yellow. Unconjugated bilirubin (i.e. fat soluble) binds to blood albumin for movement to the liver. Fat-soluble substances cannot blend into a water medium like blood without first binding to a transport protein. With the aid of two carrier proteins known as X and Y, bilirubin enters the liver, where it combines with **glucuronic acid** (which is derived from glucose) to form **bilirubin diglucuronide**. This conjugated form (i.e. water soluble) becomes a component of bile produced in the liver, and thus drains into the digestive system. Bilirubin in the colon is acted on by bacteria creating urobilinogen, which will be absorbed back into the blood and excreted in the urine. The remainder will be incorporated into the stools

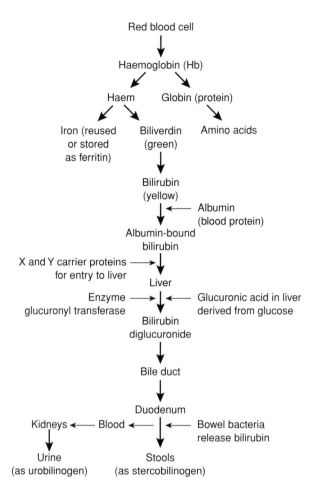

FIGURE 5.10 The natural history of bilirubin. Red cell breakdown causes the release of haemoglobin, which quickly breaks down into a haem group and the protein globin. Globin can be further reduced to amino acids; the haem group (containing iron) releases the iron, which can be stored or re-used. The remainder is biliverdin, which is green, and this is converted to yellow bilirubin. Albumin, a blood protein, binds bilirubin, and other proteins called X and Y help to transport the bilirubin to the liver. Here the enzyme glucuronyl transferase causes the bilirubin to combine with the glucuronic acid to form bilirubin diglucuronide, which becomes one component of bile. Bile arrives in the duodenum, where further conversion to bilirubin creates stercobilinogen, a component of stools. Some bilirubin is re-absorbed into the blood and filtered in the urine as urobilinogen.

(sometimes referred to as **stercobilinogen**, sterco = of the faeces). Normal urobilinogen levels in urine are small (0.09–4.23 µmol per 24 hours), but levels will increase in **jaundice**. This condition is the product of a liver that is no longer able to accept or handle bilirubin adequately (i.e. **hepatic jaundice** as in **liver failure**, **cirrhosis** or **hepatitis**) or if the bile drainage is obstructed (i.e. **post-hepatic jaundice**, caused by an impacted **biliary stone** or **pancreatic cancer**). **Pre-hepatic jaundice** can also occur when the breakdown of red cells, or **haemolysis**, is happening too quickly, as in **haemolytic anaemia**, and bilirubin is produced faster than the liver can accept. The surplus is removed by the kidney and lost in the urine, but not before the excess bilirubin colours the skin and **sclera** (the white of the eyes) yellow. Bilirubin, being not normally found in urine, will appear to make urine very dark (see p. 101) along with the raised urobilinogen. Jaundice also causes yellowing of the skin and conjunctiva.

Acid–base measurement of urine

pH is the acidity or alkalinity of a substance. It is a measure of the **hydrogen ion (H⁺)** concentration (written [pH] as square brackets means concentration of). Strong concentrations gives an acid solution (low pH 1–6) and a weak concentration gives an alkaline solution (high pH 8–14). pH 7 is neutral and is the value found in most water samples tested, especially distilled water. In urine, the hydrogen ion concentration varies according to the diet and tissue metabolism from pH 5 to 8. Hydrogen is the end waste product of energy (ATP) production by the cells, from glucose or fatty acids (see Chapter 1), also from ketone production (see p. 107) and from acids taken in the diet. Because hydrogen ions cause acidity they are potentially hazardous; they have to be transported in the blood and need to be excreted. Blood pH is critical at pH 7.4, and it must be stabilised at this value. Hydrogen ions entering the blood must be buffered then removed by the kidneys for excretion. **Buffers** are a means of 'tying up' hydrogen ions into compounds so that they are unable to contribute to the hydrogen ion concentration. This allows them to be carried safely in the blood without affecting the blood pH. Examples are bicarbonate, proteins, haemoglobin and phosphate buffers. Of these, haemoglobin (Hb) is very important for buffering hydrogen ions in the blood (Hb + H⁺ → HHb), followed by blood proteins, which have a nitrogenous component (NH_2) able to take up surplus H⁺ ($NH_2 + H^+ \rightarrow NH_3^+$), and then the bicarbonates. Bicarbonates (HCO_3^-) are filtered from the blood in the glomerulus and serve to buffer urine in the proximal tubule ($HCO_3^- + H^+ \rightarrow H_2CO_3 \rightarrow H_2O + CO_2$), where CO_2 is re-absorbed and H_2O is excreted. Phosphates (HPO_4^{2-}) are major buffers in the renal filtrate of the distal tubular cells ($HPO_4^{2-} + H^+ + Na^+ \rightarrow NaH_2PO_4$). Phosphates prevent urine from becoming too acidic or alkaline, which would otherwise damage the tract lining and cause great discomfort, especially when passing urine (**micturition**). Increased urinary pH (above pH 8, i.e. alkaline urine) occurs in **alkalosis** (high blood pH, as may occur in a vegetarian diet). It occurs naturally soon after a meal. Low urinary pH (below pH 5, i.e. acidic urine) appears in **acidosis** (low blood pH as in diabetic ketoacidosis or aspirin overdose) or after the consumption of prunes or cranberries, or as a result of starvation. Disturbance of blood pH (and thus urinary pH) can happen in various therapies that influence the fluid balance of the body. Since H^+ and K^+ share the same excretory mechanism in the distal tubule and collecting duct cells, the excretion of large quantities of K^+ (as may be the case with excessive intravenous KCl treatment or diuretic therapy) may cause retention of H^+.

Nitrites in urine

Nitrites can be tested for as an indicator of the presence of infection in the urinary tract. Nitrites are the result of the breakdown of nitrates in the urinary system. Nitrates are a component of our diet and are excreted normally in the urine. The presence of nitrites, however, indicates a bacterial infection by types of organism that are capable of producing an enzyme, **nitrate reductase**, necessary for converting nitrate to nitrite. Ninety per cent of UTIs are organisms of this type (e.g. Gram-negative bacteria such as *Escherichia coli*), and therefore the nitrite test stick is of increasing clinical importance as a quick, accurate means of detecting urinary tract infections. The remaining 10% of urinary infections include *Staphylococcus*, *Pseudomonas* species and enterococci. These are organisms that do not produce the enzyme and are therefore not sensitive to this test. Chemical stick reagent tests can often replace the more expensive laboratory tests. Urine cultures and microscopy are the largest numbers of requests made to pathology departments for laboratory examination (Valenstein 1986), and it is possible that this workload, and the cost to the health service this causes, could be reduced by incorporating some laboratory tests within the stick format

(Valenstein 1986). The nitrite and leucocyte test strips (described p. 111) are an attempt to identify those urines with infection before laboratory culture, and they therefore reduce the time and cost involved in the analysis of negative samples. The problems have centred around the accuracy of the chemical test strip, which if used routinely for the identification of urinary tact infections before laboratory cultures is thought to miss some clinically significant infections. Some authors, however, are already convinced that stick analysis of urine for infection is now accurate enough to be used to identify only those urines that need laboratory culture and analysis (Ravichandron *et al.* 1994).

Leucocytes in urine

Leucocytes of the granulocyte type (especially neutrophils) produce another enzyme, **leucocyte esterase**, that can be detected in urine. This test will identify the presence of intact and lysed granulocytes in the urine either with or without infection. The presence of leucocytes indicates an inflammation: with organisms (infection) or without (sterile).

When to test urine

Urinalysis has become a standard routine test carried out on admission to hospital and in the doctor's surgery, and it is often expected regardless of whether or not it is required for the patient's assessment. It is easy to see why these tests have become so widespread. The tests are quick, cheap, non-invasive with on-the-spot results, and they can provide a wealth of information by virtue of there being multiple tests on one stick. The alternative is laboratory analysis of urine, which is time-consuming, more expensive and on average the results take a few days to return. For reagent strip analysis, all that is required is a very small quantity of fresh urine, one stick and a few minutes of the nurse's time. If the results are recorded as NAD (nothing abnormal detected), then it is known that the renal system appears to be functioning normally, the chance of trauma is less and there is probably no diabetes, keto-acidosis, bleeding or jaundice. For these reasons, methods for putting other urine tests on a reagent strip are being considered so that the test can be ward based rather than laboratory based. The nitrite and leucocyte tests are two of the results of these initiatives; previously urinalysis for urinary tact infections took about 3 days of laboratory work for a result. Although this is still necessary to identify the organism and the antibiotic required for treatment, a quick reagent strip test that can identify the presence or absence of urinary tact infection will cut down the number of sterile specimens sent to the laboratory and in many cases provide instant reassurance to the patient. By making it possible to do a test in the clinical area the test itself becomes far less labour intensive, more cost-effective and reduces the time factor to minutes, an important point for patient comfort and recovery. No doubt other stick-mounted tests will be developed, which by reducing the laboratory input allows more laboratory time for other things.

As a standard screening device, reagent strip urinalysis can be carried out as routine almost anywhere, and certainly on admission to hospital, pre-operatively, post-operatively, and in the outpatient clinic and the accident centre, where it can be used to help eliminate trauma to the kidneys. In the community, it can be used in the doctor's surgery or in the patient's own home by visiting nurses. Being simple to use, it can also be taught to the patient to do for themselves or by the patient's carer. Chemistry has come to the aid of the health care professional and has allowed the test to be taken to the patient rather than the patient (or at least their urine) to be taken to the test.

Key points

- The functional unit of the kidney is the nephron. About one million nephrons exist in each of the two kidneys.
- Urine forms in three steps: filtration from the glomerulus, re-absorption from the convoluted tubules and secretion from the straight collecting ducts.
- Urine is formed at an average rate of 1 ml per hour.
- For accurate results, urine must be tested when fresh using the correct technique.
- Normal urine is a pale straw colour, clear with no deposits.
- On testing, normal urine should show negative results for glucose, blood, protein, ketones and bilirubin.
- Urinary pH ranges from 5 to 8 with an average about 6.
- The specific gravity measures the density of dissolved solutes in urine compared with water, normally about 1010 (water = 1000).
- Nitrite and leucocyte tests for infection or inflammatory cells in urine.
- Diuretic drugs induce a large urine output as a treatment for hypertension, oedema or cardiac failure.

References

Cook R. (1995) Urinalysis. *Nursing Standing*, 9(28): 32–35.

Cook R. (1996) Urinalysis, ensuring accurate urine testing. *Nursing Standard*, 10(45): 49–52.

Ford F. (1992) Feeling off-colour. *Nursing Times*, 88(5): 64–68.

Lloyd C. (1993) Making sense of reagent strip testing. *Nursing Times*, 89(48): 32–36.

Ravichandron D., Daltrey I., Uglow M., Johnson C. D. (1994) Urine testing for acute lower abdominal pain in adults. *British Journal of Surgery*, 81: 1459–1460.

Valenstein P. (1986) New roles for the urine dipstick. *Medical Laboratory Observer*, February, 63–66.

Walsh M. (1989) Urinalysis: a guide for students. *Nursing Standard*, 4(1): 30–31.

Wells M. (1997) Urinalysis. *Professional Nurse Study Supplement*, 13(2): S11-S13.

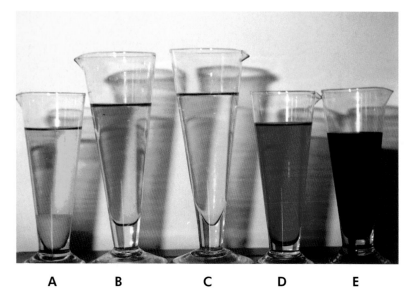

A	**B**	**C**	**D**	**E**

PLATE 1 Different colours of urine and sedimentation. A, chalky sedimentation, which may indicate the excretion of too much calcium; B, concentrated urine, as may be passed on a hot day or because of reduced fluid intake; C, dilute urine, as may be passed when fluid intake is high; D, blood in the urine (frank haematuria); E, dark urine seen in jaundice, when the urine is rich in bilirubin.

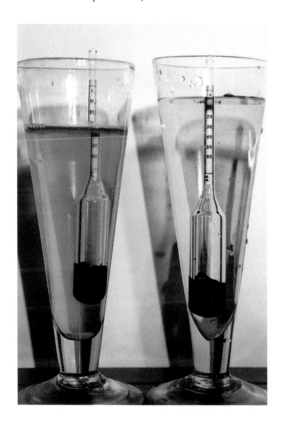

PLATE 2 Different densities of urine and specific gravity. A (left): denser (darker) urine, which indicates less water is lost through the kidneys, as occurs on a hot day and when dehydrated. B (right): dilute urine, as may be passed when fluid intake is high. Note the hydrometer (urinometer) floats lower in B than in A, and deeper urine is needed to keep the hydrometer from touching the bottom. The hydrometer is a measure of the density observed.

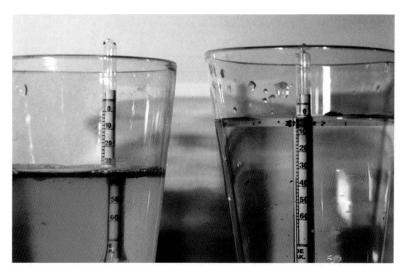

Plate 3 Different densities of urine and the hydrometer scale. A (left): denser urine that measures between 30 and 40 on the hydrometer scale (where the urine level crosses the scale). B (right): dilute urine that measures close to 0 on the scale. Zero is the specific gravity of pure water, so B is not much denser than pure water. Note that the hydrometer appears 'broken' in A owing to the different refraction (bending) of light seen through denser urine.

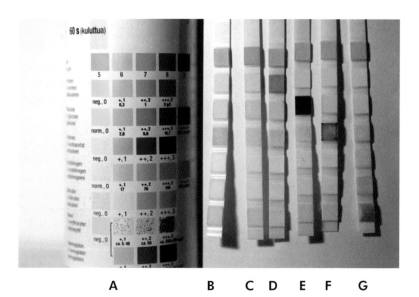

A   B   C D   E   F   G

Plate 4 Urine testing strips. A, the colour chart for comparing the colour changes seen on the strips after immersion in urine. The tests are, from top to bottom, pH (measuring the acidity or alkalinity of urine), protein, glucose, ketones, urobilinogen, bilirubin, blood and haemoglobin. B, a stick essentially normal with pH approximately 7; C, a stick with pH 5 (acidic); D, protein is present; E, large amounts of glucose; F, positive for ketones; G, positive for blood.

Chapter 6

Elimination (II): digestive observations

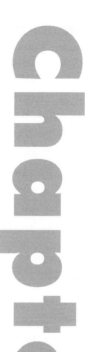

- Introduction
- Faeces
- The mechanism of defecation
- Disorders of faecal elimination
- The mechanism of vomiting
- Observations regarding vomiting
- Drugs affecting vomiting
- Nutritional observations

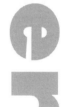

Introduction

Although generally thought of as a distasteful subject, abnormal elimination, such as diarrhoea or vomiting, indicates that changes have occurred in the patterns of physiology within the digestive system, changes of which the nurse must be aware. The presence of these phenomena alone is an important observation, but additional data can be obtained from further observation and questioning to ascertain any associated evidence. An understanding of the facts gained from observation, combined with a knowledge of the underlying pathophysiology, allows the nurse greater opportunities to make accurate decisions, for example when to involve the medical staff.

Faeces

Faeces is waste material obtained primarily from ingested food. It normally contains **fibre**, a collective term for several indigestible components of the diet that provides the bulk of the stool. Fibre is derived mostly from the plant substances in the diet, i.e. fruit and vegetables, but less is found in meats. The varieties of fibre include **cellulose**, **hemicellulose**, **pectins**, **gums** and **lignins**. These are mostly large molecular **polysaccharides** that form the walls of plant cells. These particular polysaccharides are complex carbohydrate molecules that are indigestible by any of the digestive enzymes in the small bowel (**ileum**), but some can be broken down (**catabolism**) to a certain extent by digestive bacteria present in the large bowel (**colon**). These bacteria are **commensals**, that is they survive in the human bowel without causing any harm. In fact, human bowel commensals actually produce important vitamins from their activity on bowel contents, i.e. **niacin,** which is also known as **nicotinic acid**, **thiamine**, which is **vitamin B_1,** and **vitamin K**, which we can absorb and use. Fibre has several properties; in particular, it absorbs and holds water, **electrolytes** and bile salts. Holding water makes it soft normally so that the stool is easy to pass. However, the action of the colon in absorbing water from the bowel contents prevents the faeces from being too wet normally. The absorption of electrolytes and bile salts into the fibre itself aids the elimination of these substances. **Refined foods** are those in which the fibre is largely removed or cooked sufficiently to break it down to digestible carbohydrates and provide a greater degree of nutrient efficiency with less waste material. The refining of foods, as is common in the Western diet, has resulted however in an increase in bowel disorders such as colon cancers and **diverticular disease**. The latter is a condition in which the mucous lining of the bowel is pushed through the muscular wall into pouches that can become inflamed. Clearly, fibre has a greater role to play in human digestion than was at first thought, being vital for correct bowel function and, as such, is protective against bowel disease.

The mechanism of defecation

The rectum is normally empty. Bowel wall movements push faecal matter into the rectum stretching the rectal wall. This stretching triggers the **defecation reflex** (Figure 6.1), an automatic action involving afferent sensory pathways from stretch receptors in the rectal wall to the spinal cord, and efferent motor pathways from the cord to the rectal

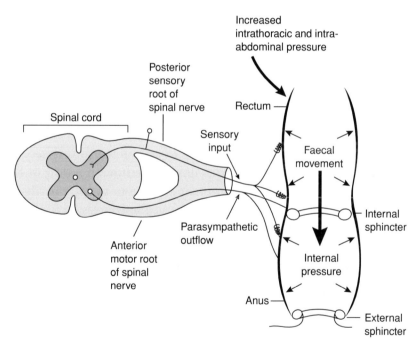

FIGURE 6.1 Physiology of defecation. Internal pressure from descending stools into the rectum stretches the rectal wall. Sensory input from stretch receptors trigger a parasympathetic output from the spinal cord which relaxes the internal sphincter and contracts smooth muscle in the bowel wall. This puts pressure on the external sphincter to open, but being voluntary skeletal muscle this sphincter opens under conscious control. Increasing intrathoracic and intra-abdominal pressure pushes the bowel contents forward.

muscles. Activation of this pathway results in the muscular walls of the sigmoid colon and rectum to contract, pushing the contents further along, and the anal sphincters to relax. Relaxation of sphincters causes them to open, and here this means opening the escape route for faeces. However, whereas the internal anal sphincter is autonomic (smooth muscle), the external requires voluntary control (skeletal muscle), thus allowing the time needed for the sphincter to be opened appropriately. It is this last aspect that is important in childhood, for control of the external sphincter is a skill that has to be learnt. Expulsion of faeces is achieved by contraction of the rectal wall, depression of the diaphragm and contraction of abdominal muscles, the last two causing an increase in the intra-abdominal pressure, aided perhaps by holding the breath. Although this is a spinal reflex, achieved by the **parasympathetic nervous system** from the sacral outflow (Figure 6.1), the medulla is involved in co-ordinating the various muscle activities. It is useful to think of the parasympathetic nervous system as being the neurological control of all three normal emptying mechanisms of the body, i.e. urination, defecation and (in males) ejaculation.

Disorders of faecal elimination

Diarrhoea

The word **rrhoea** arises at the end of several words such as diarrhoea and steatorrhoea, and it means flow. **Diarrhoea** is a flow of faeces in fluid form, since the water content is paramount and the fibre bulk is minimal. Diarrhoea has numerous causes, and nurses should make some basic observations to establish a possible **aetiology**. The nurse should observe for quantity and number of bowel evacuations that occur per day. This will give an estimate of the fluid loss the patient is experiencing, and fluid balance records may be necessary. Identification of any abnormal content, e.g. the presence of blood or mucus, is important.

Blood in the stools

Blood in the stools may be fresh and red, indicating a bleed somewhere within the colon itself. Otherwise it may be a darker red-brown (or even black, and is then called **melaena**), suggesting that the blood has undergone some degree of digestion. In this case it must come from higher in the digestive system: a bleed within the stomach or ileum.

Digestive bleeds can arise from mucosal ulcerations or growths that erode blood vessels, ruptures of varicose veins within the oesophagus or rectum, or abdominal trauma. Being a liquid itself, blood can provide the necessary water to prevent colonic contents from being converted to solid stool, and blood therefore can become thoroughly integrated with the faecal matter. Of course, heavy digestive bleeds are likely to be accompanied by other symptoms of blood loss, notably pallor, increased and weakened pulse rate, low blood pressure and even shock.

Mucus in diarrhoea

Mucus is the natural secretion of the mucous membrane and acts as a lubricant in the bowel for the passage of food and faecal content and dissolves some nutrients before it is itself re-absorbed. Mucus in diarrhoea is an indication of excessive inflammatory changes within the mucous membrane that result in overproduction of mucus. **Inflammatory bowel disease (IBD)** is a term that encompasses at least two bowel disorders, **ulcerative colitis** and **Crohn's disease**, both characterised by inflammation of the mucous lining of the bowel with blood and by mucus present in the diarrhoea.

Other causes of diarrhoea

Diarrhoea can also be caused by overstimulation of bowel movements by the parasympathetic nervous system, which promotes digestive activity. Normally, bowel contents are propelled along by waves of muscle contraction (called **peristalsis**) at a speed that allows water to be absorbed and therefore faeces to be well formed. If this rate of propulsion is speeded up (known as increased bowel **motility**), the contents reach the rectum before water is absorbed and liquid faeces results. This speeding up of peristalsis also causes the other symptom associated with diarrhoea, that of very frequent bowel evacuations and abdominal pain that occurs during peristalsis (known as **colic**). A patient suffering from a severe form of IBD, for example forty or more diarrhoea bowel evacuations in 24 hours, may sometimes experience sleep loss and severe restriction of activities. Such a patient could also experience dehydration and electrolyte imbalance and distressing pain and tenderness around the anal ring. Infections such as *Shigella*, an organism that causes **dysentery**, or food-poisoning organisms such as *Staphylococcus* or *Salmonella* can have similar effects. Non-infectious causes include the overuse of **purgatives** (or **laxatives**, see p. 120), **malabsorption syndromes**, certain foods in the diet that increase bowel propulsion, treatments like radiation therapy involving the digestive tract and even anxiety (**'nervous diarrhoea'**).

Drug-induced diarrhoea is an important cause of the problem, especially in elderly people because this group often requires more medication than younger people, and therefore they suffer more side-effects (Ratnaike and Jones 1998). **Antibiotic drugs** can cause diarrhoea as a side-effect because their activity against living organisms may also involve killing the natural colonic commensals, bacteria we need for normal bowel function. Drugs of the laxative kind fall into four main groups: the bulk-forming agents (e.g. ispaghula husk, known as Fibrogel or Isogel), the stimulants (e.g. senna, known as Senokot), the faecal softeners (e.g. oils, such as arachis oil) and the osmotic laxatives (e.g. lactulose).

Constipation

Constipation, is the failure to evacuate the bowel adequately, often totally, leading to an increasing collection of faeces in the colon. Perhaps as many as 10% of the Western population suffers varying degrees of retained bowel content, and nurses will be required to deal with the problem possibly on a daily basis. Unlike diarrhoea, constipation provides few external clues to its presence, and the nurse usually relies on a history of bowel activity over the previous few days to identify the problem. It is so important for nurses to recognise the patient who is *at risk* of constipation: notably the patient with reduced mobility, altered levels of consciousness, inadequate fluid intake or any combination of these. The case of one elderly lady illustrates this point. She was immobile, drowsy, hypothermic and not drinking well with a degree of dehydration. After several days on the ward she developed abdominal pain. Nobody on the ward knew if this lady had passed any faeces since she had been admitted. The doctors discovered she was constipated and ordered an enema, which was given by the nurses, and this solved her problem. The relatives were very pleased with the nurses actions since her pain had been relieved, but in fact the nurses has failed to recognise that this lady was at risk of constipation from the moment of admission. Her pain was *preventable*, not just *curable*, by the identification of her risk status, by the monitoring of her bowel movements and by the correction of her dehydration. In some patients improvements in their mobility also contributes to the prevention of constipation, as well as the many other complications of immobility.

One bowel evacuation each 24 hours is the average, but considerable variation does occur, with some individuals claiming that bowel evacuations of only once or twice per week is normal for them. Others may pass faeces more that once a day. What *is* abnormal is a total absence of any bowel evacuation, and what *may* be abnormal is a significant change in a person's bowel habit, especially if this change is persistent. If once a day is normal for an individual, then 3 days without evacuation is a potential for constipation. Additional signs to aid the nurses diagnosis of constipation include the presence or absence of **anorexia** (loss of appetite), abdominal pain and distension, nausea and confusion. This last symptom is particularly important in elderly people, when the brain becomes especially susceptible to the toxic effects of constipation, i.e. waste products that are normally excreted are re-absorbed into the blood; confusion as a result of constipation must be identified as families can think that their elderly relative is becoming demented when all that is required is an enema. Diet is also important to note, since a lack of oral fluid or fibre in the diet is an important factor leading to constipation (Cooper and Wade 1997). Lack of exercise, especially complete immobility, reduces bowel movement, which, in turn, causes the contents to remain longer in the colon. During this longer stay in the colon more and more water is absorbed from the contents, which then get drier and harder to propel and evacuate. Total obstruction of the bowel with hard, solid faeces can follow on from this in some extreme cases, made worse by any condition that narrows the bowel lumen, like new growths. Drugs that have a constipating side-effect include **morphine** and its derivatives. High dosage, as in the management of some terminal disorders, may cause this unwelcome effect, which then requires additional management. Assessing the risk of constipation requires keen observation of diet and fluid input, mobility, attempts at defecation, abdominal pain and mental alertness, and these are sometimes put together in risk assessment scales, which may be useful in some clinical areas (Duffy and Zernike 1997). Elderly people are always said to be at highest risk because of reduced mobility and a decline in the health status of the bowel with age (Towers and Burgio 1994).

Stomas

A **stoma** is an artificial opening in the bowel to allow the excretion of bowel contents into a collection bag on the abdominal wall when normal defecation is not possible. Stomas are made into the ileum (**ileostomy**) or colon (**colostomy**) depending on the nature of the problem. Stomas are sometimes used in the management of bowel cancers, ulcerative colitis, diverticular disease or after permanent **bowel resection** (removal of part of the bowel). A colostomy opening made into the *proximal* half of the colon (on the right side of abdomen) will, at first, result in a more liquid stool than an opening into the *distal* half of the colon (on the left side of the abdomen). This is due to the water extraction function of the colon. The proximal half contains liquid stools from the small intestines, whereas the distal half contains stools that have travelled nearly the entire length of the bowel and are therefore much drier. Stoma bags require changing, which the patient can often do themselves after recovery from surgery and after being taught about their stoma. Observation is important during the changing procedure, when the stoma itself should be examined for a healthy red (the natural colour of mucous membrane that is well supplied with blood) with no bleeding. Pallor or cyanosis (blue coloration) may indicate reduced blood supply, which can cause complications, and must be reported to the doctor. The skin around the stoma must be inspected for soreness and inflammation, any broken areas and infection. This is important since some collection devices work by sticking to the skin, and this could become problematic. The bag contents are observed for the same constituents as faeces, i.e. for diarrhoea, blood, bile or mucus, and also colour and quantity. Some drugs may affect the function of stomas or change the colour of the bag contents. These drugs include laxatives and antacids (both of which are best avoided for most stoma patients unless prescribed and monitored carefully). **Narrow-spectrum antibiotics** are preferable to **broad-spectrum antibiotics** when such drugs are necessary, since narrow spectrum means they will have less effect on the normal bowel commensals with less risk of diarrhoea. Diarrhoea in a stoma patient is very difficult to manage since it requires numerous changes of the collection bag, which disrupts normal daily activities and results in complications of the skin at the stoma site. Skin irritation and breakdown around the stoma is particularly unfortunate and should be avoided if possible. The broad-spectrum antibiotics, like penicillin, can not only cause diarrhoea but directly irritate the skin at the stoma site. Antibiotics can also change the faeces to a grey-green colour. Other colour changes caused by drugs include iron (black), tetracycline (red), heparin (pink or red), indomethacin (green) and aspirin (pink or red). This last drug, aspirin, is acidic and therefore may cause mucosal and skin irritation at the stoma site. It also contributes to anticoagulation of blood, i.e. helps to stop blood clotting and promotes bleeding, and is therefore best avoided for these reasons. Stoma care is a specialist nursing subject and nurse practitioners train specifically in this subject. Stoma patients will be referred to the care of such a specialist nurse, who should be consulted on all matters concerning these patients.

The mechanism of vomiting

Vomiting can be regarded generally as a normal physiological response to an abnormal condition affecting either the digestive system or its neurological control. Stomach, and sometimes bowel, contents are driven the wrong way up the oesophagus back into the mouth. This usually only happens as a result of a pathological state, and accurate observations can provide important clues about the nature of this pathology.

The brain stem medullary **vomit reflex centre** co-ordinates what is a relatively complex process involving a range of different stimuli (Figure 6.2). Also in the brain, and closely associated with the vomit centre, is the chemoreceptor trigger zone. This is in the floor of the fourth ventricle (within an area called the **area postrema**), and this receives impulses from chemical stimuli in the blood. These chemicals include various drugs (e.g. cytotoxic agents) and other toxins from perhaps food or infectious organisms. Such stimulation of the **chemoreceptor trigger zone** causes stimulation of the vomit reflex centre, and vomiting can then occur. The chemoreceptor trigger zone also receives impulses from the **cerebellum**, part of the brain that co-ordinates muscle activity and balance. The cerebellum obtains sensory information on balance (**vestibular** information) from the semicircular canals in both ears via the vestibular branch of the eighth cranial nerve (the **vestibulocochlear nerve**). These canals register changes in balance and head movement as nerve impulses that are transmitted first to the **vestibular nuclei** in the medulla, then to the cerebellum (Figure 6.3). Any disturbing movements or upsets in balance, as in motion sickness, can produce adverse nerve impulses that pass through the vestibular nuclei, the cerebellum and on to the chemoreceptor trigger zone. From here the vomit reflex centre is stimulated and vomiting occurs. A disease that causes vomiting via this route is **Ménière's disease**, a chronic disorder

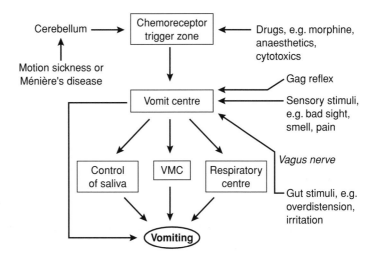

Figure 6.2 Stimulation of the vomit centre is often via the chemoreceptor trigger zone, which itself is stimulated by motion or drugs, or sometimes directly by bad sensory stimuli (e.g. an unpleasant smell or sight) or by vagal stimuli from the gut. The vomit centre output is via the vasomotor centre (VMC), which influences the blood pressure, via the respiratory centre, which regulates breathing throughout vomiting; the vomit centre controls saliva production.

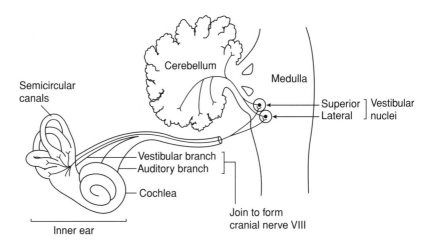

Figure 6.3 Vestibular stimulation of the cerebellum. Impulses from the semicircular canals of the inner ear pass via the vestibulocochlear nerve (cranial nerve VIII) to the vestibular nuclei of the medulla and then on to the cerebellum.

of the inner ear where the amount of the fluid called endolymph becomes excessive. This causes sudden attacks of **vertigo** (dizziness), nausea and vomiting, progressive deafness and **tinnitus** (continued internal sounds in the ear). It is interesting that the word vertigo has become commonly associated with dizziness caused by heights. However, the word simply means dizziness; it is not especially related to heights, and in reality people can suffer from vertigo at any height, often at ground level.

Some stimuli can cause vomiting without affecting the chemoreceptor trigger zone, i.e. affecting the vomit reflex centre directly. These include the **gag reflex**, a feeling of retching when the back of the tongue is touched with a finger or tongue depressor. Bad sights or smells stimulate the vomit reflex centre via the **cerebral cortex**, our conscious part of the brain, and stimuli from the digestive tract itself, such as overdistension or inflammatory irritation, arrive at the vomit centre via the **vagus nerve** (the tenth cranial nerve) (Figure 6.4).

The result of initiating activation of the vomit reflex centre is to first induce **nausea**, a feeling of sickness without actual vomiting, followed by retching and then finally vomiting. The person will inhale deeply as peristalsis is reversed. **Peristalsis** is the propulsive intermittent waves of smooth muscle contraction that pass along the bowel to push the contents forwards. Reversal of the direction of this contraction wave ensures that the digestive contents will be driven towards the mouth during vomiting. Just as with swallowing, the airway must be protected against inhalation during vomiting. Inhalation of vomit would involve not only obstructing the airway, but gastric acid and digestive enzymes would severely damage the delicate lung tissues and death would occur. To prevent this, the glottis is closed by lowering the epiglottis and raising the hyoid bone and larynx. The **glottis** is the narrowest part of the airway opening and is found inside the larynx. The **epiglottis** is a flap of cartilage above the glottis that acts as a lid for the glottis by folding downwards at the same time as the **larynx** (voice box) is raised. In this way the glottis is closed and vomit cannot pass into the lungs. The **soft palate** is raised to close the **nasopharynx**, the passage from the nose to the throat, to prevent vomit entering the nose. If this is not achieved properly vomit may come from the nasal passages as well as the mouth. The top opening into the stomach is dilated (called the **cardiac sphincter** because it is close to the heart), and the lower opening (the **pyloric sphincter**) is closed. The gastric muscles (smooth type) and abdominal muscles (skeletal type) both contract forcing the stomach

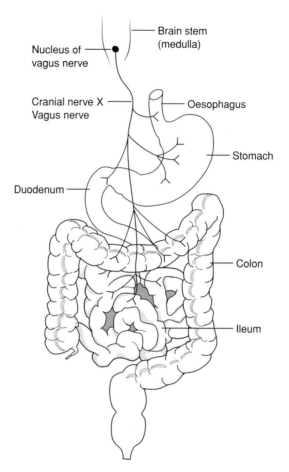

FIGURE 6.4 Vagus innervation of the digestive tract. The vagus (cranial nerve X) is the primary visceral sensory nerve. Branches to the stomach increase gastric acidity and the parasympathetic component promotes digestion generally.

contents upwards towards the mouth. The **diaphragm** (skeletal muscle) also flattens to aid in this process, helping to increase the intra-abdominal pressure. The process leaves the person a little breathless because energy is used (the generation of which requires oxygen, see Chapter 1) and breathing has been temporarily suspended. It is also accompanied and preceded by increases in both salivation and heart rate, the onset of pallor, sweating, pupillary dilation and distress, much of which is caused by **sympathetic nerve** stimulation of the sweat glands, the heart and the pupils.

Nausea, which is simply feeling sick, acts as an early warning that vomiting may happen. It is an unpleasant sensation that may persist alone or quickly result in the act of vomiting. It can occur under all the same pathological conditions that cause vomiting. However, nausea, and sometimes vomiting, can occur in non-pathological conditions, e.g. they are often features of early pregnancy (i.e. **morning sickness**). This is probably due to hormonal changes occurring at that time, especially the introduction of hormones from the placenta, such as **human chorionic gonadotrophic hormon**e (**hCG**), or hormones from the **corpus luteum**, and the gradual decline in these pregnancy-related hormones is associated with the relief of sickness (Coutts 1998).

Approximately one-quarter of people coming into hospital for treatment of cancer feel nauseated on arrival, before the therapy has begun. It can happen before second or subsequent treatments where side-effects experienced from the first treatment are anticipated. This is termed **anticipatory nausea and vomiting** (**ANV**) and can sometimes be relieved or prevented in susceptible patients (Banks 1991, Blasco 1994).

Observations regarding vomiting

The nurse needs to take into account how much is vomited, what the contents are and when does vomiting occur. The quantity is important because the gastric volume is limited, and the stomach may not have been full originally. Vomiting should stop once the stomach has been emptied if this was the purpose of the phenomenon. When this happens it suggests that a cause lies within the stomach itself or its contents. But, if vomiting persists beyond this point, it is likely to become unproductive once the stomach is empty, or produce only small volumes of gastrointestinal fluid. **Retching** is an attempt to vomit but with no gastric or duodenal content produced. At this point it is possible to say that the process of vomiting is not solely to empty the stomach but is caused by factors outside the digestive system continuously stimulating the vomit reflex centre in the brain. This in turn is affecting what is quite possibly a normal stomach.

In all cases, the nurse should ascertain some basic facts by asking questions, when possible, e.g. how long has the vomiting persisted? The nurse should also ask if the vomiting is associated with:

1 pain (e.g. abdominal or migraine);
2 the intake of food in general, or specific foods, drugs or alcohol;
3 exposure to motion, as in spinning round, sea or travel sickness;
4 exposure to obnoxious substances or emotionally disturbing experiences, e.g. the sight of blood, someone else vomiting or a foul smell; and
5 persistent coughing. This is a phenomenon mostly seen in children, in whom prolonged coughing may stimulate the vomit reflex centre. The cough and vomit centres both occur close together in the medulla, part of the brain stem.

How long the vomiting has persisted is vital because prolonged vomiting results in fluid and electrolyte losses leading to imbalance and of course various degrees of malnutrition. This is especially so for children, who will become ill rapidly if the fluid and electrolyte imbalance is not corrected quickly and vomiting is not brought under control. In addition, the nurse needs to observe the product of the vomiting to identify whether it is food (digested or not), blood, bile or other gastrointestinal fluids.

Food in vomit

Food when vomited indicates that the time span between eating and vomiting is relatively short, i.e. within 4 hours of each other, and generally the shorter the time span the less digestion has occurred. In this case, either the stomach cannot tolerate the food, or the food itself causes a vomit reaction. The former happens often as a result of infection or inflammation of the stomach (**gastritis**), or if the food was accompanied by large quantities of alcohol, or due to the inability of the stomach to pass food into the bowel because of an obstruction. One example of obstruction is **pyloric stenosis**, as seen in young children. This is a restriction of the flow of gastric contents through a tight or closed pyloric sphincter. Pyloric stenosis can be associated with **projectile vomiting**, when peristalsis attempts to force food through the obstruction but actually ejects it. Bowel obstructions are also caused by new growths (**neoplasms**) or compression of the bowel by abdominal muscle contractions, as seen in **strangulated hernias**, both conditions found in the older adult. Some degree of obstruction can occur in istortions of the bowel like **intussusception** (telescoping of the bowel) or **volvulus** (twisting of the bowel), both of these being conditions found usually in children.

The latter situation, where the food itself causes the vomiting occurs as a result of infections or toxins in the food (**food poisoning**). A number of different organisms cause food poisoning of varying degrees, some more dangerous than others, e.g. *Clostridium botulinum*, the cause of **botulism**. This is a rare but fatal form of food poisoning often contracted after eating contaminated canned meat products. Such contamination results from failure of the can-sealing process, or ruptured seals on cans during transport. All the seals at the joints in the metal of canned meats should be inspected before purchase, and any breaks in these joints reported to the shop staff. A less dangerous, yet very unpleasant, food poisoning is caused by *Staphylococcus aureus*, usually implanted on food by those preparing the food. This gives 24 hours of vomiting and diarrhoea, leaving the person feeling debilitated and very unwell.

Blood in vomit

Blood appears in different forms in vomit, depending on where the bleeding is occurring. Fresh bright-red blood in the vomit means it has not been in the stomach for very long, perhaps only minutes, and may indicate a possible gastric bleed, known as a **haematemesis**, from an ulceration or **neoplasm** (new growth). However, swallowed blood, often from an **epistaxis** (nose bleed), can be vomited back since the acidic stomach cannot tolerate large quantities of blood. This is a good reason for holding the head forward when treating nose bleeds, to prevent posterior bleeding, which will otherwise be swallowed and cause vomiting. Vomiting blood can continue for sometime, i.e. until the patient collapses from shock, and requires urgent intervention. Sudden massive quantities of vomited blood are sometimes seen in ruptured **oesophageal varices**, varicose veins of the lower oesophagus caused by congestion of hepatic portal venous blood as a result of obstructive liver diseases (Figure 6.5). An important cause of liver obstruction is **cirrhosis**, a gradual loss of liver cells that are replaced by scar tissue, and which is usually accompanied by **hepatic failure**.

Blood that has been in the stomach for an hour or more before being vomited has been subject to changes caused by digestion and the hydrochloric acid conditions. In this case it is described as **coffee grounds**, a reference to its appearance. This type of bleeding indicates low-grade blood loss, which the stomach can tolerate for a while, possibly from an ulceration.

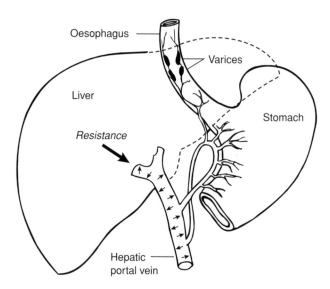

FIGURE 6.5 Oesophageal varices caused by portal hypertension. High blood pressure inside the portal vein (shown by small arrows inside the vessel) is due to some resistance to blood flow within the liver, often the result of liver disease. Back flow of blood to the lower end of the oesophagus causes venous dilatations, which can rupture and bleed severely.

Bile in vomit

Bile and other gastrointestinal fluids do occasionally appear in vomit, especially if persistent vomiting has emptied the stomach and has forced duodenal or even ileal contents up into the mouth. About 500 ml of bile comes from the liver each day into the duodenum (see Chapter 1), and it gives a strong unpleasant alkaline burning taste in the mouth when vomited. The digestive system as a whole produces 7 l of fluid secreted into the bowel lumen over 24 hours, which consists of saliva (1.5 l), gastric juice (2 l), pancreatic juice (1.5 l), bile (0.5 l) and intestinal juice (1.5 l), which contains digestive enzymes, mucus, cells and other products. Normally most of this is re-absorbed (6.5 l from the small intestines and 350 ml from the colon per day), but it can be vomited as a watery fluid, usually seen after heavy or persistent bouts of vomiting.

Faeces in vomit

Vary rarely it is possible to vomit faeces. This happens only in the event of a severe bowel obstruction that has persisted for quite sometime, when any form of bowel evacuation has stopped. The actual time involved may vary from one patient to another. Under these conditions it becomes necessary to empty the bowel as much as possible while supporting fluid and electrolyte balance before urgent surgical intervention.

Drugs affecting vomiting

Vomiting can be caused or prevented by various drugs. Some **emetics**, such as **apomorphine** (derived from **morphine**), are drugs that can cause nausea and vomiting by stimulating receptors on the chemoreceptor trigger zone (see Figure 6.2). The list of drugs that act in this way includes **cytotoxic agents** (used in cancer therapy), some of the **opiate analgesics** that act on the brain stem (such as morphine), some **anaesthetics** and **ipecacuanha**, a substance that is both a digestive irritant and a chemoreceptor trigger zone stimulant. This has been used with good effect in emergency departments to cause vomiting in children suspected of an accidental oral overdose of drugs. **Pilocarpine** is a drug that can cause vomiting by stimulating the cerebellum directly, thus bypassing the chemoreceptor trigger zone.

Drugs with the opposite effect are the antiemetics, which prevent vomiting in several ways. **Anticholinergics** (e.g. **hyoscine**) block stimuli from the vestibular system and are therefore useful in the treatment of motion sickness. Try checking the ingredients of several brands of travel sickness tablets to see which ones contain hyoscine. The side-effects are sometime troublesome, notably a dry mouth, blurred vision and drowsiness. Drowsiness is dangerous if driving, and a warning against combining these drugs with driving should be on the pack. The **antihistamines** are also used in motion sickness therapy; they are less effective than hyoscine but produce less side-effects. They include cyclizine, promethazine and dimenhydrinate. These drugs block receptor sites for **histamine** (the H_1 **receptor**), but it is not clear how they prevent sickness. **Cannabinoids**, such as the drug **nabilone**, act on the chemoreceptor trigger zone and are useful in treating sickness during cytotoxic therapy, but they do cause drowsiness, dizziness and a dry mouth. The **dopamine antagonists** work by blocking the dopamine receptors (type D_2 **receptors**) in the area postrema, reducing the chemoreceptor trigger zone stimulation of the vomit reflex centre. They are therefore less useful in treating motion sickness. Included in this group are thiethylperazine and the non-phenothiazines metoclopramide and domperidone. Metoclopramide can also act on the stomach, promoting its emptying via the normal pyloric route. The side-effects are sedation, **hypotension** (low blood pressure) and some problems of movement involving the **extra-pyramidal tract system** of the brain.

Nutritional observations

Observing the nutritional status of patients involves a number of specific assessments that together will give insight into the dietary needs of the patient. Nutritional assessment often starts with the diet, not just the current diet but the dietary history, which is especially important on admission. Nutrition should be ascertained from what the patient and relatives say about the patient's eating habits at home, and whether or not they have been eating a **balanced diet**. This means a diet containing all the necessary daily portions of protein, carbohydrate, fats, fluids and fibre. Vitamin and mineral intake is harder to judge, and if deficiency is suspected this would require investigation.

The patient is weighed and any previous weight loss identified is noted. Daily weighing recorded on a weight chart will permit further weight loss to be detected. Weight loss may mean **dehydration** in the first instance if the patient does not drink enough. Additional weight loss can involve body fat losses, followed later by protein reduction in the form of **muscle wasting**. However, not all weight loss is due to poor dietary intake. Some terminal conditions cause changes in the body metabolism that result in reduced body bulk. The term **cachexia** refers to this moribund state of metabolic malnutrition found in the terminally ill (see Chapter 1).

While in hospital, the simple observations are often the best, e.g.

1 ensuring that the patient is able to eat;
2 ensuring that the patient eats adequately and drinks enough to sustain fluid balance;
3 observing the patient's mouth daily to assess cleanliness and identify any oral infections that cause pain on eating and reduce the appetite; and
4 checking that false teeth are clean, well-fitting and that the patient uses them.

Deficiencies of all kinds in the diet do occur in hospitals for many reasons. The patient can be **nil by mouth (NBM)** for quite some time, and dextrose or saline intravenous infusions provide very few nutrients. Vomiting (see p. 123) and pain will block the appetite, and digestive disorders may make feeding or digestion difficult. Some patients, especially the frail, may suffer a mild degree of **kwashiorkor**, a lack of protein accompanied by stress. Inadequate food intake and the stress of admission, pain, investigations and surgery all contribute to this condition (Figure 6.6). It is important that the nurse recognises that vitamin and mineral deficiencies, dehydration and a lack of fibre can also occur in hospitals (Edwards 1998).

Key points

- Diarrhoea and vomiting are indications that changes have occurred in the patterns of physiology within the digestive system.

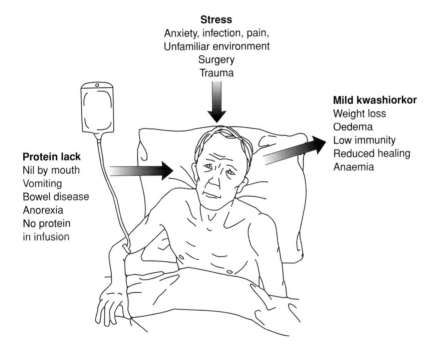

Stress
Anxiety, infection, pain,
Unfamiliar environment
Surgery
Trauma

Mild kwashiorkor
Weight loss
Oedema
Low immunity
Reduced healing
Anaemia

Protein lack
Nil by mouth
Vomiting
Bowel disease
Anorexia
No protein
in infusion

FIGURE 6.6 Mild kwashiorkor in hospital patients. The two basic conditions of kwashiorkor (protein lack and stress) can be present in a hospital environment. A lack of protein can be caused by anorexia, nil by mouth, continued vomiting and the absence of protein in standard intravenous therapies. Stress is caused by the removal of the patient to an unfamiliar environment, pain, fear, investigations, surgery and trauma. Nurses should be observant for signs of this condition, weight loss, oedema and reduced capacity to fight infections, in the most vulnerable, e.g. elderly people.

- Fibre has an important role to play in human digestion, being vital for correct bowel function and protection against bowel disease.
- Blood in the stools may indicate a bleed somewhere within the colon if fresh, or a bleed within the stomach or ileum if darker.
- Mucus in diarrhoea is an indication of excessive inflammatory changes within the mucous membrane that result in overproduction of mucus, as in inflammatory bowel disease.
- Diarrhoea can be caused by excessive bowel movements that can occur in bowel infections or food poisoning, the overuse of laxatives, malabsorption syndromes or treatments like radiation therapy.
- Signs of constipation include anorexia, abdominal pain, distension, nausea and confusion.
- Lack of fluid or fibre in the diet and lack of exercise are important factors leading to constipation.
- A stoma is an artificial opening in the bowel. Stomas open into the ileum (ileostomy) or colon (colostomy).
- In the event of vomiting, the nurse should check how long it has persisted, whether the vomiting is associated with any pain, food intake, drugs, alcohol, exposure to motion, obnoxious substances or an emotionally disturbing experience or whether there is any persistent coughing.
- Nurses should observe and report any food, blood, bile or faeces in vomit.
- Prolonged vomiting results in fluid and electrolyte losses, especially in children, who will become ill rapidly if the fluid and electrolyte imbalance is not corrected quickly and vomiting is not brought under control.
- Emetics are drugs that can cause nausea and vomiting, and the antiemetics prevent vomiting.
- It is important that the nurse recognises that protein, vitamin and mineral deficiencies, dehydration and a lack of fibre can occur in hospital patients.

References

Banks C. (1991) Alleviating anticipatory vomiting. *Nursing Times*, 87: 42–43.

Blasco T. (1994) Anticipatory nausea and vomiting: are psychological factors adequately investigated? *British Journal of Clinical Psychology*, 33(1): 85–100.

Cooper J. W. and Wade W. E. (1997) Constipation in the geriatric patient. *Journal of Geriatric Drug Therapy*, 12(1): 49–69.

Coutts A. (1998) The 'minor' problems of pregnancy: a review. *Professional Care of Mother & Child*, 8(4): 95–97.

Duffy J. and Zernike W. (1997) Development of a constipation risk assessment scale. *International Journal of Nursing Practice*, 3(4): 260–263.

Edwards S. L. (1998) Malnutrition in hospital patients: where does it come from? *British Journal of Nursing*, 7(16): 954–974.

Ratnaike R. N. and Jones T. E. (1998) Mechanisms of drug-induced diarrhoea in the elderly. *Drugs-Aging*, 13(3): 245–253.

Towers A. L. and Burgio K. L. (1994) Constipation in the elderly: Influence of dietary, psychological and physiological factors. *Journal of the American Geriatrics Society*, 42(7): 701–706.

Chapter 7

Neurological observations (I): consciousness

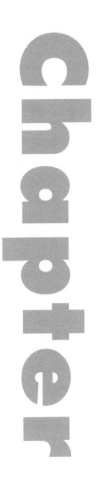

- Introduction
- The cerebral cortex
- Observations of consciousness
- Major causes of unconsciousness
- The anaesthetic drugs
- Key points

Introduction

To science, consciousness is a problem, referred to as *the hard problem*, simply because it cannot be explained. There is no current understanding how brain cells can create a subjective experience like consciousness, i.e. trying to integrate the chemical activity of the cell with a concept of reality. But this understanding is so important to the medical and nursing professions, and there are some known facts. The brain area involved in consciousness is the **cerebral cortex**; and it is worth thinking of this large area as *the conscious brain*. An area called the **prefrontal cortex**, part of the **frontal lobe**, is the primary centre for consciousness; the site of the *self* and many higher intellectual functions (Carter 1998). All other parts of the brain function at an unconscious (or subconscious) level, although many supply the cortex with essential information that makes consciousness possible. What subconscious means is that these other areas work without the individual's awareness or control; so these are qualities of consciousness. First, awareness of the environment involves communication of environmental stimuli to the brain via the **sensory nervous system** and the **special senses**, such as vision and hearing. This is important since the brain is almost entirely encased within the skull, cut off from the outside world, and can only appreciate this world through sensory stimuli. It also means awareness of your own thoughts, known as the process of **cognition** (= mental activity). Second, control suggests some form of meaningful interaction with the environment, mostly through the **motor nervous system**, based on an understanding of the environment and what that interaction will achieve. Sensory *input*, cognitive *processing* and motor *output* can be likened to the functions of a computer, the brain being the most advanced form of computer available. Awareness and control are lost in patients who are unconscious, i.e. the computer is *switched off*.

The cerebral cortex

When viewed from the side, the front or the top, the largest part of the human brain seen is the cerebral cortex (Figure 7.1). As *the conscious brain*, the cerebral cortex is responsible for the awareness and control identified above as being the components of consciousness. The cortex is made up of nerve cells called **neurones** that have multiplied by **mitosis** (cell division) many millions of times during the embryonic development of each individual. After birth, however, all neuronal cell

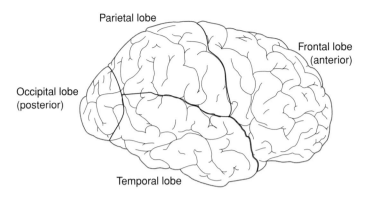

Parietal lobe

Frontal lobe
(anterior)

Occipital lobe
(posterior)

Temporal lobe

FIGURE 7.1 The cerebral cortex from the right side showing the major lobes.

division effectively stops, so the cell numbers never increase again. This means that neurones lost during life cannot be replaced. The rest of the brain is also made of neurones, but they never achieve consciousness, and it is this unique function of the cerebral cortex cells that is so puzzling. Neurones have a cell body and a long process, called the **axon**, extending for varying distances away from the body (Figure 7.2). **Dendrites** are shorter cell body processes connecting cells together. Dendrites are afferent (= *towards*) because they convey impulses towards the cell body; axons are efferent (= *away from*) because they convey impulses away from the cell body. The axons are mostly **myelinated**, i.e. covered by a fat (lipid) layer, the **myelin sheath**, the purpose of which is to speed up nerve impulse transmission from about 2 metres per second (unmyelinated) to as much as 120 metres per second (myelinated). In the cerebral cortex, this myelin layer is formed by cells called **oligodendrocytes** during embryonic development. Oligo-dendrocytes are just one type of a collection of support cells called **neuroglia** (often shortened to **glial cells**). Glial cells do not convey nerve impulses; instead, they provide other structural or chemical functions that are essential for brain activity. Considering the human brain has 10^{10} neurones, which are just 10% of the brain cells present, the other 90% are neuroglia, how many glial cells are there? Of this vast number, most are astrocytes (named after their star shape), which have vital chemical and nutritional roles to perform in the brain. Myelin sheaths, being made of fat from oligodendrocytes, makes the axons appear white, whereas cell bodies, being free from myelin appear grey. Hence, **grey matter** consists of cell bodies packed together, as on the surface of the cortex, whereas **white matter** consists of axons packed together as they extend deeper into the brain (Figure 7.3). Just think of

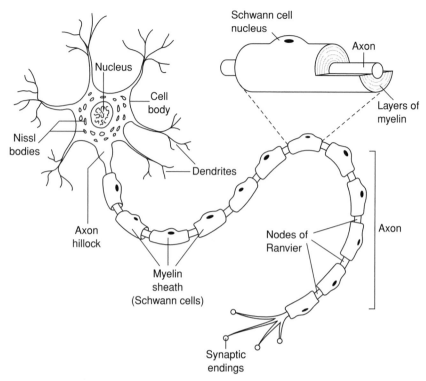

Figure 7.2 The neurone. The cell body shows a nucleus surrounded by Nissl bodies. The axon starts at the axon hillock and terminates at the synaptic endings. Myelin covers the axon in segments with gaps between, called the nodes of Ranvier. An enlarged myelin segment is shown. Myelin is laid down in layers by cells called Schwann cells.

a helium balloon seller at a fair; the balloons are all together up high (the cell bodies of the cerebral cortex grey matter), whereas the balloon strings are all extending down, parallel to each other, into the balloon seller's hand (the myelinated axons forming white matter extending downwards from the cortex).

The cerebral cortex has a major division, the **longitudinal fissure** along the midline running from front to back (antero-posteriorly). This separates the cortex into two halves, the left and right hemispheres, which are connected deeper down by the **corpus callosum**. It is through the corpus callosum that communication between the two hemispheres can occur. Each hemisphere is further divided by fissures into lobes given the same names as the bones that overly them. Thus the frontal lobe is anterior to both the **parietal** and the **temporal lobes**, separated from the **parietal lobe** by the **fissure of Rolando** (or **central sulcus**)

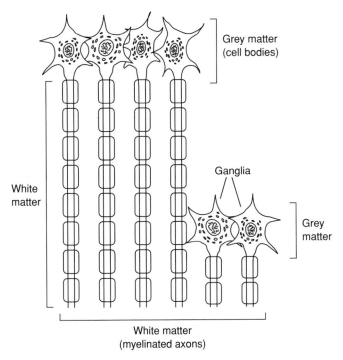

FIGURE 7.3 Neurones in clusters form grey matter (cell bodies) and white matter (axons). Ganglia are cell bodies (patches of grey matter) separated from the main group of cell bodies.

and separate from the **temporal lobe** by the **fissure of Sylvius**. Posterior to all these, at the back of the cortex is the **occipital lobe**. A **sulcus** (pl. **sulci**) is a gully across the brain surface between two ridges (or **gyrus**, pl. **gyri**), causing the surface to be folded to increase the total area. In this way more grey matter can be packed into the limited skull cavity. Fissures are usually deeper divisions than sulci and mark the boundaries of the lobes.

The cells of the cerebral cortex are arranged in a strict pattern according to function; thus it becomes possible to map the brain surface (Figure 7.4). It is not surprising that these functional areas are all related to the activities we identified with consciousness, i.e. *control* (motor function of the frontal lobe areas), *awareness* (sensory functions of the parietal, temporal and occipital lobe areas, and cognition of the frontal lobe and other **association areas**). Association areas exist between the main functional areas of the cortex and are essential for making sense of the sensory stimuli arriving at the cortex. They contain memory banks developed from previous sensory experience that are used for

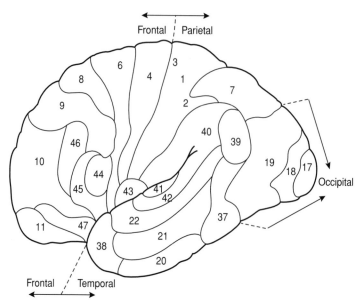

FIGURE 7.4 Map of the left cerebral cortex according to cell function. Each area has a Brodmann number.

comparing with new stimuli. An example would be that if we hear a bell ring we know this is a bell because we have heard previous bells ringing and can therefore make that association. A new-born child, hearing a bell for the first time does not know what it is since there is no previous experience or knowledge of this sound. Association areas must learn these sensory stimulatory patterns and store them as memories for future use if the individual is to make sense of the world. This is one reason why the human brain is unique in taking a longer time than any other species to mature, i.e. up to 20 years or more. There are important association areas working with:

1 the parietal sensory area, which receives sensations from the body (**somatic sensations**; soma = body);
2 the occipital sensory area, which receives visual sensations from the eye (the **visual cortex**); and
3 the temporal sensory areas receiving sensations of hearing (the **auditory cortex**) (Figure 7.4).

Even within the main specialised functional areas of the **motor cortex** (frontal lobe) and **sensory cortex** (parietal lobe), the cells are carefully arranged in a layout that matches the body plan (Figure 7.5). Although

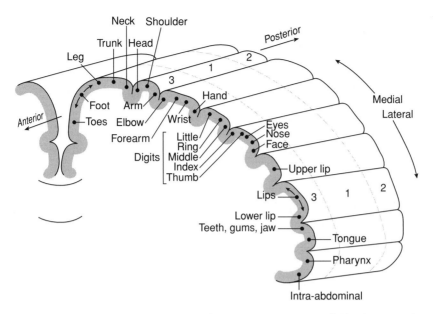

Figure 7.5 The sensory cortex (Brodmann areas 1, 2 and 3), showing the layout of cells according to the areas of the body that they receive transmissions from. Notice the large areas involved in sensation of the lips (a very sensitive area) and the large areas for the fingers and the hands compared with the feet and toes.

the appropriate motor cortex cells control the muscles they are ultimately connected to, the delivery of somatic sensations to the relevant cells in the sensory cortex is more complex. Sensations coming into the brain from the body must first pass to the **thalamus,** a sensory relay station deeper within the brain that sorts the sensations and sends them on to the correct cerebral cells. Consider the sensory cortex as a massive company, each cell being one office. In comes a telephone call (sensory stimulus) destined for one specific office. The call must first go to an exchange (the thalamus) that connects the caller to the correct office within the company. It is important that this sorting process takes place since, for example, cells in the sensory cortex that specialise in the toes would not be interested in sensations arising from the ears, just as the occupants of one office would not be interested in taking calls destined for elsewhere. The thalamus is therefore the brain's *server* (as on a computer network), directing the *e-mails* (stimuli) to the correct *terminal computer* (sensory cell). What is amazing is that nature designed and operated computers with server systems some four million years or so before the first computer was invented.

Neurones connect to each other through **synapses**, microscopic gaps between one axon and what lies beyond, which could be a cell body or dendrites, or another axon (Figure 7.6). Some neurones may have up to 100,000 synaptic connections each with other neurones. These tiny gaps require a bridging chemical, called a **neurotransmitter**, to fill the gaps during the passage of an impulse, and thus cause changes, like a new impulse, beyond the synapse (i.e. in the **post-synaptic membrane**). There are many different neurotransmitters, but the main chemical in the cerebral cortex is **glutamate**. Glutamate is considered to be the neurotransmitter of consciousness, although it does function elsewhere in the brain in some subconscious areas. Glutamate is

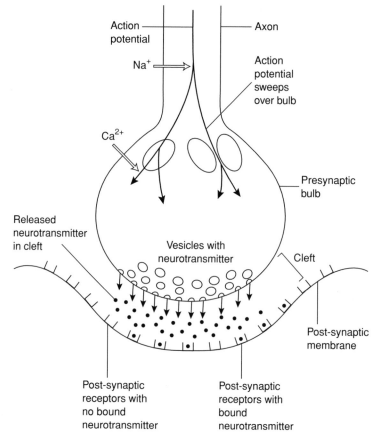

FIGURE 7.6 The synapse. As the action sweeps down the axon to the presynaptic bulb, the influxing ion changes from sodium (Na^+) to calcium (Ca^{2+}). The vesicles release a neurotransmitter into the cleft and the chemical binds to receptor sites on the post-synaptic membrane. A bound neurotransmitter will have an effect on the cell beyond the post-synaptic membrane.

excitatory in almost every site it is used, i.e. it generates a new increase in activity when released at the synapse, like the accelerator system of a car when used. Glutamate is produced as part of a chemical cycle that also generates another neurotransmitter called **GABA** (short for **gamma-aminobutyric acid**) (Figure 7.7). This chemical is largely **inhibitory** because by filling the synapse it blocks any changes in the post-synaptic membrane and therefore acts like a brake in the car in slowing brain activity. It should not be surprising that the brain has acceleratory and braking abilities like a car, because this allows the brain to operate at a modest level most of the time (like an average car speed), with the option of increasing or decreasing brain activity (going faster or slower) as the need arises. By carefully regulating the chemical cycle that produces both the excitatory and inhibitory neurotransmitters, the brain can fine tune glutamate or GABA production to meet its activity needs.

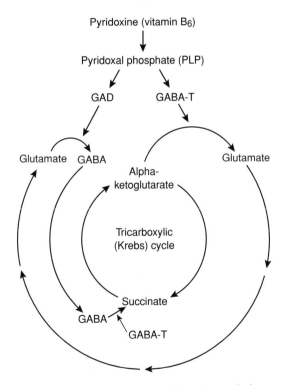

FIGURE 7.7 The gamma-aminobutyric acid (GABA) and glutamate (glutamic acid) cycle. The Krebs cycle (Figure 1.1) provides alpha-ketoglutarate as the starting point for glutamate, which returns to the Krebs cycle as GABA. The enzymes are GABA transaminase (GABA-T) and glutamic acid decarboxylase (GAD). Vitamin B_6 (pyridoxine) is important for these enzymes to function.

Observations of consciousness

It is not enough to consider a person either conscious or unconscious since there are various degrees of consciousness and changes in the levels of consciousness. It is useful to consider a spectrum from fully conscious at one end to a deep state of unconsciousness, known as **coma**, at the other. The various points on this spectrum are the **altered states of consciousness** (Figure 7.8). Notice that **sleep** does not appear on the same spectrum. Sleep is an altogether different state and should not be confused with unconsciousness. Sleep is distinguished from unconsciousness by several characteristics, notably that sleep is a natural body requirement during which the subject is rousable. Also, sleep has a typical pattern of brain activity that can be observed using an electroencephalograph, a machine for measuring and displaying the electrical output of the brain which produces an **electroencephalogram (EEG)**.

It becomes important to assess the level of consciousness in a patient for two reasons. First, the point the patient occupies on the spectrum of consciousness is important since this has a bearing on the management of the patient's condition and prospects for a successful recovery (**prognosis**). Second, it is very important to know whether the patient is moving along the spectrum, either by regaining consciousness or more urgently to know whether the patient is deteriorating by going into coma. But assessing consciousness is difficult because the patient may be unresponsive, and only close observation of specific signs can provide any evidence of the conscious state.

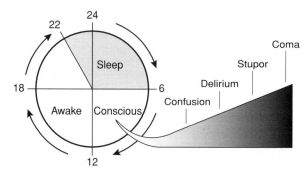

FIGURE 7.8 The consciousness–coma continuum and the sleep–wake cycle. The sleep–wake cycle is normal, but the coma continuum is due to pathology.

The **coma scale** is a series of such specific signs that can be assessed and will give some evidence of the conscious state and any changes in it. The specific signs are assessed by the nurse delivering a sensory stimulus to the patient and then observing the response. The grade recorded on the coma scale will depend on the patient's best response to that stimulus. Auditory stimuli are usually tried first. These are sounds beginning with normal speaking, e.g. asking the patient a question (e.g. *what is your name?*). If no response then give a louder command (e.g. *open your eyes*) or a clap of the hands. Such stimuli enter the brain via the **vestibulo-cochlear nerve** (**cranial nerve VIII**, previously known as the **auditory nerve**) and directly excite neurones of the auditory cortex within the temporal lobe (see p. 140 and Figure 7.4). If no response to auditory signals is noted then **tactile stimuli** are tried. These are touch-related somatic sensations (e.g. *gently shaking their arm*), which pass via **spinal nerves** to the **spinal cord** then on to the brain stem and upwards to the thalamus, which relays the stimulus onto the appropriate part of the parietal lobe's somatic sensory cortex. Thus speech and touch pass by different routes to different areas of the cerebral cortex. Just as we increased the auditory stimulus by raising the volume from speech to command, so we can increase the somatic stimulus from touch to pain. Almost every conscious person responds to **painful stimuli** in some form or another; it is a powerful stimulus of cerebral cortex function. However, pain is associated with injury, and it is very important to use a method of pain application that causes no tissue damage. Traditionally, rubbing the sternum with the knuckles of a clenched fist has been used, but this practice should stop since bleeding has often occurred causing large haematomas and ultimately extensive bruising over the front of the chest. It is better to apply pressure to the finger and toe nails, which are themselves dead tissue and therefore will not be damaged. The response to pain is *motor*, i.e. a reaction from the frontal lobe's motor cortex causing the muscles to move the limbs in some manner. Even a verbal response to pain is motor in origin, albeit from the brain's specialised motor speech area (called **Broca's area**), again in the frontal lobe, but such a reaction would probably mean that the patient was fully conscious. The somatic motor responses can be called **purposeful responses** if they show limb withdrawal from the pain, or attempts to push the nurse's hand away (i.e. they show signs of trying to stop the pain, so the pain is registering as conscious). The limb movements may cross the body's midline. **Non-purposeful responses** are limb movements without any attempt to stop the pain or withdraw from it, and do not cross the midline, whereas **unresponsive** is a feature of the deepest comas. Pain is interesting because it is handled by the nervous system somewhat differently from all other stimuli. All somatic pain passes into the spinal cord and then onto the thalamus, but both the cord and the thalamus have their own ways of managing pain. The spinal cord has a **reflex arc**, which is either a direct or an indirect connection between the sensory neurones carrying the pain stimulus and the motor neurones taking impulses to the muscles. The painful stimulus flashes across the cord from back (sensory) to front (motor) and causes an impulse to rapidly pass to the muscle, the contraction of which pulls the body part away from the source of the pain. It all happens in milliseconds (i.e. thousandths of a second)! Obviously, being a spinal cord reflex, this happens at a subconscious level, having nothing to do with the level of consciousness higher up in the cerebral cortex. Consequently, some limb responses to pain will be affected, or modified, by the presence of a spinal reflex response, although higher centres do influence the reflex arc to some extent. It may not always be possible to determine how much of a limb response to pain is cortical and how much is spinal; this is one of the problems of choosing pain as a stimulus. The thalamus is the other player in our story. Earlier it was noted that the cerebral cortex was the conscious brain, with all other areas functioning at subconscious levels. This is true of the thalamus except for pain, which registers as conscious at the thalamic level. Therefore, it is reasonable to say that the application of painful stimuli is more a test of thalamic *conscious* function than of cerebral cortex *conscious* function. By the time we arrive at pain in our test sequence most of the motor response to that pain is likely to be thalamic in origin, the previous verbal and tactile stimuli having already identified the cerebral cortex as unresponsive.

Brain stem reflexes

Being the upward extension of the spinal cord, the brain stem not only houses the vital centres of cardiac, blood pressure and respiratory function, it is also the home of several reflexes other than pain. The **pupillary reflex**, which controls the size of the pupils and their reaction to light, and the **corneal reflex**, which causes the lids to close sharply when the surface of the eyeball is touched, will both be examined in Chapter 8. The **gag reflex** occurs when a stimulus is applied to the back of the throat and this induces a sensation of retching (wanting to vomit; see Chapter 6). Such a stimulus would be a spatula or a finger placed at the back of the tongue. It is similar to the spinal cord's pain reflex arc: a sensory input passes to the vomit centre in the medulla, which triggers the motor response from the muscles of the throat and upper digestive tract; the muscles then carry out the reaction. Like all reflexes it is protective, attempting to prevent objects from obstructing the vital passages from the mouth to the digestive system and helping to keep the airway clear at the same time.

Coma scales

A coma scale is a means of identifying and recording levels of consciousness in the patient. Terminology has been developed to help in the process of positioning a patient on the consciousness spectrum using specific criteria or symptoms that may be present in any combination (see Figure 7.8; all modified from Hickey 1997):

> **Fully conscious**: awake, alert, orientated in time and place, understands spoken words, reads written words, expresses ideas verbally.

Then the altered states of consciousness:

> **Confusion**: disorientated in time, place and person; memory lapses; short attention spans; difficulty in following instructions; possibly hallucinations or false perceptions; agitation and bewilderment.
> **Lethargy**: orientated but very slow in motor activity and speech, low level of mental activity, high accident risk.
> **Obtundation**: very drowsy, arousable when stimulated, verbal responses very limited, attempts to follow only very simple commands, high accident risk.
> **Stupor**: generally unresponsive except to vigorous verbal or touch stimuli, attempts at eye opening or incomprehensible sounds may be the only response, responds to pain, minimal spontaneous movements, high accident risk.
> **Coma**: no response to verbal or touch stimuli, no verbal sounds, response to pain stimuli as follows:
> **Light coma**: purposeful withdrawal from pain, gag, corneal and pupillary reflexes intact.
> **Medium coma**: non-purposeful responses to pain, variable brain stem reflex responses, some being absent.

Deep coma: unresponsive to pain, brain stem reflexes absent.

Several coma scales have been developed but the **Glasgow coma scale** has been the most widely adopted (Figure 7.9). This assessment defines coma as three conditions: the patient is unable to open the eyes, is unable to obey commands and is unable to speak. Eye opening, motor response to both verbal commands and painful stimuli and the

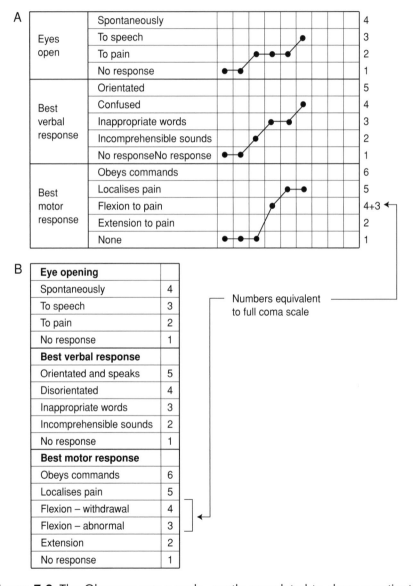

FIGURE 7.9 The Glasgow coma scale, partly completed to show a patient regaining consciousness.

ability to speak are the specific signs adopted for assessment (Figure 7.9). The patient is assessed by applying various stimuli and observing for a response in these areas. Reliability between different observers is good, making this a valid tool for the universal assessment of consciousness (Juarez and Lyons 1995).

The **Rancho Los Amigos** scale (Table 7.1), named after the Rancho Los Amigos Hospital, uses levels of cognitive function to assess consciousness: from level 1 (fully unconscious) to level 8 (fully alert) (Hagen *et al.* 1972, Malkmus and Stenderup 1974).

Major causes of unconsciousness

Epilepsy

An abnormal pattern of electrical activity that renders the brain unconscious is called **epilepsy**. The affected person may go through a convulsive phase (or have a fit), but this is not always the case, since various types of epilepsy are known (Table 7.2). The cause is often a

TABLE 7.1 The Rancho Los Amigos assessment scale

Level	Response	Appearance
I	None	Comatosed
II	Generalised	Responds to deep pain. Limited, delayed gross body movements
III	Localised	Responds directly to the stimulus; inconsistent delayed responses
IV	Confused Agitated	Heightened state of activity, confused responses, bizarre behaviour
V	Confused Inappropriate Non-agitated	Responds to simple commands, responses non-purposeful, inappropriate verbal responses
VI	Confused Appropriate	Appropriate responses to pain, can follow simple directions
VII	Automatic Appropriate	Orientated in familiar surroundings, automative behaviour patterns
VIII	Purposeful Appropriate	Alert, orientated, shows reasonable memory and learning capacity

small area of damaged or disturbed brain tissue, the **epileptogenic focus**, which may or may not be detectable and may or may not be operable. In any case, the focus acts as a trigger by causing an abnormal burst of electrical impulses both sideways (laterally) into adjacent cells and down the axons to all parts lower down. This is because the focus is overactive and can discharge impulses very easily. Part of the reason for this hyperactivity is a lack of GABA at the focus (see p. 145), which results in a loss of the inhibitory (braking) system, and the accelerator glutamate goes out of control (like a car with no brakes). Other chemical changes at the focus cause this area to become very excitable, such as an abnormal influx of calcium (Ca^{2+}) into the focal cells and disturbances

TABLE 7.2 The various types of epilepsy

Grand mal	Major convulsive fit in several phases (see Figure 7.11). Complete loss of consciousness with no memory of the event
Petit mal (absences)	Minor fit. Brief episode of staring vacantly (loss of touch with reality) during which objects held are dropped. Recovery in seconds.
Jacksonian	Twitching in one point in the body spreading to all other parts and causing loss of consciousness
Focal	Twitching in one point in the body (e.g. mouth or digit) without spread or loss of consciousness
Psychomotor	Sudden disturbance of behaviour with perhaps hallucinations. Temporal lobe epilepsy is one form
Myoclonic	Sudden involuntary muscle jerking occurring like a shock, often in the arms of known epileptics
Post-traumatic	After severe brain injury. It involves all epileptic types except petit mal
Status epilepticus	Repeated epileptic fits, often one after another, before consciousness is regained and lasting for many hours

to glucose and protein metabolism. Impulses travelling down normal cell axons move in one direction only, away from the cell body, called **orthodromic** flow, but **antidromic** (backward flow of the impulse along the axon from the synapse towards the cell body) is seen in abnormal conditions such as the epileptogenic focus. Each time the axonal impulse returns to the cell body it regenerates a new orthodromic impulse that travels down the axon. This cycle of events is repeated many times during a convulsion causing the rhythmic thrashing of the limbs as each new impulse from this cycle passes out to the muscles (Figure 7.10). The lateral spread of the abnormal burst of impulses across the brain surface causes the other cerebral cells to stop all conscious activity, and the person goes unconscious for the duration of the fit, perhaps about 3–5 minutes. Breathing, the heart cycle and blood pressure remain, since they are not conscious activities and are controlled by brain areas lower down in the brain stem. The course of events during a convulsion (or grand mal fit) involves several brief moments of

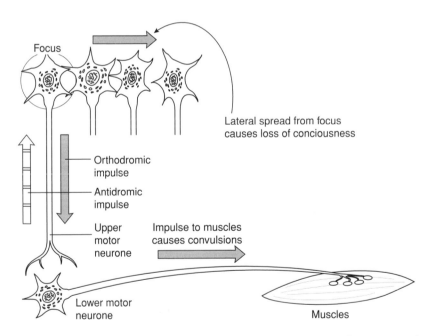

FIGURE 7.10 Events that occur during a fit. The epileptogenic focus spreads abnormal impulses laterally to cause the cerebral surface cells to lose consciousness. Impulses travelling in a normal direction down the focal axon (orthodromic) not only cause impulses to pass out to the muscles (creating seizures) but return abnormal impulses back to the focus (antidromic) as part of an impulse loop up and down the focal axon.

collapse, rigidity (the tonic phase), convulsion (the clonic phase) and full recovery (Figure 7.11). Minor fits (often called petit mal or vacancies) involve a short period of staring into space with fumbling followed by complete recovery. This is not unconsciousness as such but a kind of twilight state in which the brain is incapable of all normal conscious responses and goes into *pause* or *standby* mode. Post-epileptic twilight states can be a serious complication of a convulsion, when the patient can wander aimlessly for hours or days not knowing who or where they are.

Strokes

Strokes, or **cerebrovascular accidents** (**CVAs**) are sudden, usually unpredictable, disruptions to the blood supply to the brain. The blood carries essential oxygen and glucose to the neurones and carries away the wastes of cellular metabolism, and sudden loss of these functions can cause neurones to cease functioning. In the case of the cerebral cortex neurones this causes unconsciousness. The disruptions come in two forms: bleeding into the brain itself (**intracerebral bleed**) and sudden obstruction of the blood vessels leading to the brain (**cerebral thrombosis** or **embolus**).

The blood supply to the brain begins as blood leaves the left side of the heart via the aorta (see Chapter 2). A series of arteries branch off

	Stage	Notes
1	**Aura**	A warning of impending fit. Not always present or recognised. May take the form of flashing lights or other hallucinations.
2	**Tonic**	Lasts up to 30 seconds. Full muscle tone causes gross rigidity, including respiratory muscles, causing breathing to stop.
3	**Clonic**	Lasts up to 45 seconds or so. The convulsion phase, with gross twitching and thrashing of limbs. Breathing is spontaneous.
4	**Recovery**	Clonic convulsion stops and the patient 'sleeps' off the effects for up to 15 minutes or so. Should waken with no memory of the event.

FIGURE 7.11 Stages of grand mal seizure.

from the aorta carrying blood upwards to the head (Figure 7.12). The **brachiocephalic** and **common carotid** arteries distribute blood towards the neck; the internal carotid arteries take blood up to the **circle of Willis** in the base of the brain (Figure 7.13). Blood also arrives there from the vertebral arteries, branches of the **subclavian** arteries, that pass up through the cervical (neck) vertebrae (hence vertebral). The bilateral nature of these arterial systems means that the circle of Willis has four blood supplies (two vertebral and two internal carotid arteries) but there are six main arteries going out of the circle. These are also bilateral pairs, the two **posterior**, two **middle** and two **anterior** cerebral arteries. The circle of Willis is therefore the major blood distribution point for the entire brain.

Strokes often occur as a result of one or both of two factors: either the systemic blood pressure is too high (**systemic hypertension**, see

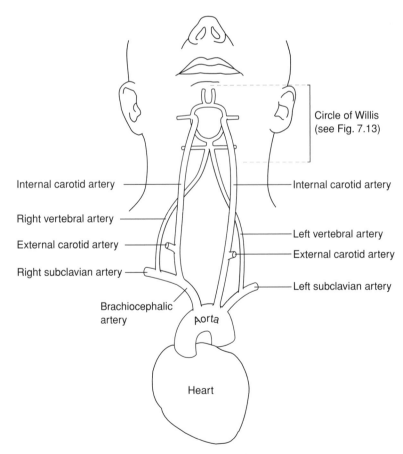

FIGURE 7.12 The blood supply to the brain from the heart.

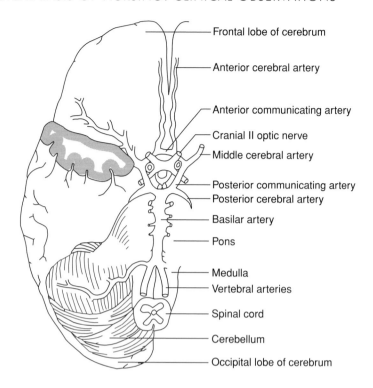

Frontal lobe of cerebrum

Anterior cerebral artery

Anterior communicating artery

Cranial II optic nerve

Middle cerebral artery

Posterior communicating artery
Posterior cerebral artery

Basilar artery

Pons

Medulla
Vertebral arteries

Spinal cord

Cerebellum

Occipital lobe of cerebrum

FIGURE 7.13 The arteries of the circle of Willis distributing blood to the brain.

Chapter 2) or arterial disease, such as arteriosclerosis, narrows the vessels and leads to **thrombosis** (blood clot formation in the cerebral arteries) or **emboli** (blood clots from elsewhere in the circulation blocking the artery). The sudden loss of blood supply causes areas of the brain to cease functioning with the loss of neurones: these areas become necrotic (dead) areas, or **cerebral infarcts** (similar to myocardial infarcts in Chapter 2). In either case, bleeding or obstruction, the effect is rather similar: sudden collapse, varying degrees of altered consciousness, including sometimes coma, severe head pain if the patient is conscious, weakness (**hemiparesis**) or paralysis (**hemiplegia**) often experienced down one side and sometimes other signs like loss of speech (**aphasia**). The signs depend entirely on where the CVA has occurred in the brain, how big the lesion is and what neurones and pathways are affected. Signs include hemiplegia (see Chapter 8) and the degree of unconsciousness. If a small area of cerebral cortex is involved in the lesion, consciousness may be retained throughout or return quickly if lost. Alternatively, large areas of cortex involved may mean prolonged coma from which the patient may never recover. Some patients suffer brain damage to the point where they die soon after the event. Recovery is also dependent on the degree of brain damage sustained. Some survivors who regain consciousness may make a full recovery, whereas others may be left with some **neurological deficit**, i.e. permanent symptoms such as one-sided weakness or speech loss, that they must learn to overcome.

Head injury

Unconsciousness in head injury is caused by shaking of the brain (known as **concussion**), damage to the brain or pressure on the brain. The difference between them is critical, i.e. the difference between full recovery (associated with pressure), partial or no recovery (associated with brain damage). Because the brain is a soft organ inside a hard bony skull, it can suffer the *jelly in a tin* effect when the head is struck. Imagine a ready-to-eat jelly placed in a tin with the lid on. If the tin is dropped from only waist height, the tin will survive more or less intact. But will the jelly? Head injuries are either a **deceleration trauma** (the head is moving but suddenly stops as it hits an immovable object) or an **acceleration trauma** (the head is stationary but is caused to move violently when struck by a fast moving object). In either case the brain movement is always slightly behind the skull movement, i.e. the skull stops suddenly but the brain carries on briefly and collides with the inside of the skull, or the skull moves suddenly and the brain lags behind and again collides with the skull. The first collision causes an injury to one part of the brain (e.g. at the front), followed by an *equal but opposite force* causing the brain to move in the opposite direction, creating a second injury directly opposite to the first (e.g. at the back), known as the **contracoup injury** (see Figure 7.14). The problem is that the top surface of the brain, i.e. the surface exposed to the inside of the skull, is the cerebral cortex: *the conscious brain*. So in either scenario, consciousness is likely to suffer first and probably most severely. Some protection to this surface is afforded by the **meninges,** which cover the surface of the brain and cord (collectively called the **central nervous system**, or **CNS**), and by the jacket of watery fluid within the meninges (the **cerebrospinal fluid**, or CSF) (Figure 7.15). The meninges are three coverings: from the inner to the outer layers they are the **pia mater**, the **arachnoid mater** and beneath the skull the **dura mater**. A small dry space, the **subdural space**, exists between the dura mater

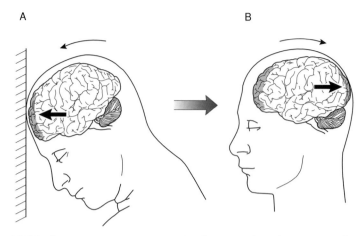

Figure 7.14 Contracoup trauma to the brain in head injury. A, the initial injury to the front of the brain when the head is thrown forward and hits a solid object; B, the secondary injury.

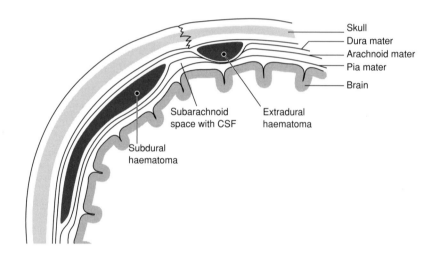

Figure 7.15 The subdural and the extradural haematomas. CSF, cerebrospinal fluid.

and the arachnoid mater below, but a larger CSF-filled space, the **subarachnoid space**, between the arachnoid mater and the pia mater below provides most of the cushioning effect around the brain. CSF is produced within the **ventricles** of the brain; it circulates around the brain and cord and is returned to the blood via the **arachnoid villi** extending from the arachnoid mater. Therefore this fluid is constantly being renewed, and a relatively constant pressure of CSF must be maintained. The hardness and roundness of the skull, plus the CSF cushion, all help to prevent brain injury during minor head collisions, like the many small head bumps children sustain with no ill effects. It takes a much harder blow to the skull, as is often a feature of injuries sustained while travelling at speed, to cause the involvement of consciousness. This demonstrates the need for external protection, i.e. helmets, plus seat belts and head rests, to prevent deceleration injury for various high-risk forms of transport.

The bony box we called the skull has a limited internal space, most of which is filled with the brain. This and the blood and CSF volumes circulating the brain cause an internal pressure within the skull, known as the **intracranial pressure** (or **ICP**), which is normally anything up to 15 mmHg. About 80% of this pressure is caused by the brain, and the remaining 20% is shared between the blood and CSF volumes. **Raised intracranial pressure** (or **RICP**), i.e. any pressure persistently sustained over 20 mmHg, is caused by anything that abnormally demands space inside the skull; a **space-occupying lesion** (or **SOL**). SOLs can be many things, such as brain tumours, excessive CSF volume (called **hydrocephalus**) and bleeding inside the skull from trauma. After brain shaking (**concussion**, see p. 157), small bleeds into the cerebral cortex may occur (brain bruising, or **contusion**); the blood lost may build up if bleeding continues and puts pressure on the brain (**compression**). The process leading to RICP is often continuous, and the casualty deteriorates with loss of consciousness. Where the bleeding occurs inside the skull is important; the most common sites associated with head injuries being the **extradural haematoma** (blood between the dura and the skull) or the **subdural haematoma** (blood in the subdural space, see p. 158 and Figure 7.15). When we discussed the meninges and the spaces between them there was no mention of an extradural space; in fact the space has to be created by the lesion, which must therefore be a high-pressure bleed, i.e. an arterial bleed (for example in the **middle meningeal artery**). This kind of injury is rarer than the venous bleed that causes the subdural haematoma, (i.e. four subdural bleeds to every extradural bleed), and extradural bleeds are even rarer in the elderly, for the dura slowly fuses onto the skull with increasing age making the creation of an extradural space almost impossible. The main differences, apart from the site and blood vessel involved, is speed of onset of symptoms. The extradural haematoma is *rapid*, i.e. life-threatening symptoms can occur within a few minutes, compared with the *slower* subdural haematoma, which causes problems over several hours or even days. This indicates two things:

1 The need for a 24-hour stay in hospital for head injuries to exclude the extradural haematoma; if the subdural develops at home after that there is time to get the patient back to hospital.
2 The need for continuous observation since the patient may deteriorate rapidly and die if vital symptoms of an extradural are missed.

The symptoms are those of RICP, and they fall into two categories:

1 **General symptoms**: those that indicate the presence of RICP but give no clue to the exact site of the pressure on the brain.
2 **Local** (or **focal**) **symptoms**: those that indicate both the presence and the site of pressure on the brain.

General symptoms are **headache** (which is worse on wakening), **nausea, vomiting, slow pulse rate (bradycardia)** and **raised blood pressure** (both of which may occur late as the patient deteriorates and should not be relied on), **altered state of consciousness** (see p. 149 and Figure 7.8), **blurred vision, respiratory irregularities** and **papilloedema** (see Chapter 8, p. 185). The focal symptoms are **unilateral, ipsilateral fixed dilated pupil** followed later by **bilateral fixed dilated pupils, nystagmus** and **visual field defects** (see Chapter 8, p. 171), **fits** (see p. 151), **aphasia** (loss of speech), **ataxia, hemiparesis** and/or **hemiplegia** (see Chapter 9, p. 206) and **specific sensory losses**. These symptoms will develop at different speeds depending on many factors, as indicated here for extradural and subdural haematomas, including which blood vessel is bleeding, the location of the bleed on the brain and the brain's compensatory mechanism. This **compensatory mechanism** allows for a certain increase in SOL size without undue change in the ICP (see Figure 7.16). As the SOL grows the pressure it exerts is *absorbed* at first by a *reduction* in both the volume of blood entering the skull and the volume of CSF produced. Remember, these two account for 20% of the ICP (see p. 159), and this percentage could drop to accommodate the growing SOL. This compensation only lasts for a while, after which the ICP will rise sharply (see Figure 7.16) since the SOL is now big enough to put pressure on the brain, which cannot reduce any of its 80% ICP value. This is the critical point, the change from compensation to decompensation, where the resultant RICP may kill the patient if this is not noticed urgently. Increasing RICP will displace the brain, forcing it downwards and/or sideways, referred to

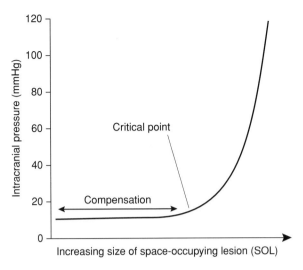

FIGURE 7.16 The sudden rise in the intracranial pressure occurs when the brain compensatory mechanism fails. This critical point must be watched for very carefully.

as **herniation** of the brain structures, with associated tearing of membranes and crushing of nerves. As the brain stem is forced downwards it impacts on the **foramen magnum**, the large opening in the base of the skull through which the spinal cord emerges. This impaction blocks the flow of CSF through the opening from brain to cord and back, and it puts pressure on the vital centres of the brain stem: the cardiac and vasomotor centres (see Chapter 2), and the respiratory centre (see Chapter 4). This is a life-threatening situation, called **coning**, and is far better avoided by accurate observation than cured. The treatment for RICP is generally a surgical opening made into the skull, called a **burr hole**, to let the haematoma out, and in the case of an extradural it may be necessary to perform this *before* the patient is taken to theatre. This vital procedure, combined with accurate neurological observation, can save the patient's life.

Other causes of loss of consciousness

Many other causes of unconsciousness exist. A group of student nurses was asked to put together a list of causes, and between them they identified more than fifteen. The list was then passed to several trained nurses, who raised the total to twenty-six. Finally, a number of doctors were asked for their contribution, and the list grew to nearly forty causes.

This illustrates just how vulnerable consciousness is to instabilities in both the internal environment of the brain and the external environment we live in, yet we take consciousness so much for granted. We do not notice it until we lose it. Here are a few important examples of causes of unconsciousness:

1 Lack of oxygen, either in the air or through strangulation, choking, drowning or airway obstruction.
2 Various poisons and toxins, such as the toxin that causes **tetanus** from the bacterium ***Clostridium tetani***, which lives in soil and infects soil-contaminated wounds.
3 Central nervous system infections, such as **meningitis** (inflammation of the meninges) or **encephalitis** (inflammation of the brain substance).
4 Intoxication by alcohol or drug abuse or overdosage.
5 Electric shock.
6 Loss of blood pressure, temporarily as in **fainting** (or **apoplexy**), or more profound as in severe shock.
7 Metabolic disorders such as **diabetes** (see Chapter 4), where both high and low blood sugar levels induce coma in response to instability in the blood insulin level.

Fainting is possibly the most common cause of unconsciousness; the one most people may suffer or encounter. The temporary drop in blood pressure causes a transient loss of blood supply to the brain, which then goes unconscious. It is usually temporary because it tends to treat itself. The original problem is caused by the brain being above the heart, which has the job of pumping blood *uphill*, against gravity, to the brain. This requires a good arterial blood pressure and therefore considerable heart pumping power, and if the left ventricle fails to deliver this blood the brain suffers. However, it is somewhat self-treating because fainting causes the person to collapse and this puts the brain *in line* with the heart, and the pressure required to supply blood to the brain is much less. In short, fainting does away with gravity. Now the left ventricle can happily supply blood to the brain at the new lower pressure, and the brain recovers. Of course, the fall can cause problems, and the casualty must remain flat until the ventricular pressure is high enough to supply the brain in the upright position. When asked, *'Under what circumstances could fainting be the cause of death?'* one student answered *'If you faint on the edge of a cliff.'* The real answer is when the person faints while pinned in an upright position, i.e. unable to fall to the ground, such as standing in a tightly packed train on a long, hot journey. The drop in blood pressure results in the blood being unable to flow uphill to reach the brain.

The anaesthetic drugs

Currently it is not possible to say exactly how many anaesthetic drugs create unconsciousness. The benzodiazepines, like Valium, and the barbiturates, such as phenobarbitone, can induce unconsciousness in sufficient dosage. These work by binding to specific GABA receptors and enhance the inhibitory (or braking) effect of GABA, thus effectively shutting down brain activity. Other anaesthetics are less well understood, but they do appear to suppress excitation of the cerebral cortex without affecting nerve conduction. Lipid solubility is a common feature of these drugs and correlates well with their anaesthetic properties, i.e. the more lipid soluble the greater is their power of anaesthesia. Perhaps they get incorporated into cortical neurone cell membranes, which are themselves lipid based. Distortion of these membranes by the drugs may disrupt ionic movement across the membrane and cause the neurone to fail temporarily.

Key points

- The cerebral cortex, particularly the prefrontal cortex, is the conscious brain.
- Awareness of the environment and control of activities are qualities of consciousness.
- The cortex is made up of nerve cells called neurones.
- Neurones have a cell body with dendrites and an axon that is often myelinated.
- Neuroglia (or glial cells) provide structural or chemical functions important for neurone activity.
- Grey matter is cell bodies packed together and white matter is axons packed together.
- Neurones connect to each other through synapses. These tiny gaps require a neurotransmitter, the most important of which for consciousness is glutamate.
- Another neurotransmitter is GABA (gamma-aminobutyric acid), which inhibits nerve impulses.

- The left and right hemispheres of the cortex are further divided into lobes given the same names as the skull bones: the frontal, parietal, temporal and occipital lobes.
- Association areas between the main functional areas of the cortex are essential for making sense of the sensory stimuli arriving at the cortex.
- The motor cortex is in the frontal lobe, the sensory cortex is in the parietal lobe. The cells are carefully arranged in a layout that matches the body plan.
- Sensations coming into the brain from the body must first pass to the thalamus, a sensory relay station that sends sensations on to the correct part of the cerebral cortex.
- Consciousness can be considered as a spectrum, from fully conscious at one end to coma at the other. The various points on this spectrum are the altered states of consciousness.
- Painful stimuli are achieved by applying pressure to the finger and toe nails, which are dead tissue and therefore will not be damaged. The response to pain is motor, i.e. limb movements.
- Purposeful responses are signs of trying to stop painful stimuli; non-purposeful responses are limb movements without any attempt to stop painful stimuli.
- The Glasgow coma scale is the most widely adopted. This defines coma as unable to open the eyes, unable to obey commands and unable to speak.
- The cause of epilepsy can be a small area of damaged or disturbed brain tissue, the epileptogenic focus.
- The grand mal fit involves collapse, tonic rigidity, clonic convulsions and then full recovery. Minor fits (petit mal or vacancies) are short periods of aimless staring with fumbling followed by complete recovery.
- Strokes, or cerebrovascular accidents (CVAs), are sudden, unpredictable disruptions to the blood supply to the brain, bleeding into the brain itself (intracerebral bleed) or sudden arterial obstruction (cerebral thrombosis or embolus).
- Unconsciousness in head injury is caused by shaking of the brain (concussion), damage or pressure on the brain. The difference between them means full recovery (associated with pressure), partial or no recovery (associated with brain damage).

- Some protection to the brain is afforded by the meninges, the pia mater next to the brain, the arachnoid mater and beneath the skull, the dura mater, and by the cerebrospinal fluid, or CSF. The subdural space exists between the dura mater and the arachnoid mater below.
- The development of an extradural haematoma is rapid, within minutes, compared with the slower subdural haematoma, which takes several hours or days.
- The symptoms of raised intracranial pressure (RICP) are general (those that indicate RICP but no clue to the site of the pressure) or focal (those that indicate both RICP and the site of pressure). A slow pulse rate and raised blood pressure may occur late and should not be relied on.
- Coning, i.e. death by impacting the medulla through the foramen magnum, is avoidable with accurate observation.
- Fainting is a common cause of unconsciousness caused by a temporary drop in blood pressure with loss of blood supply to the brain. It is somewhat self-treating because collapse puts the brain level with the heart, and the pressure required to supply blood to the brain is much less. If a person faints while pinned in an upright position, i.e. unable to fall, it could be fatal.

References

Carter R. (1998) *Mapping the Mind*. Weidenfeld and Nicolson, London.

Hagen C., Malkmus M. and Durham P. (1972) http://www.neuroskills.com/~cns/tbi/rancho.html

Hickey J. (1997) *The Clinical Practice of Neurological and Neurosurgical Nursing*, 4th edn. Lippincott, Philadelphia.

Juarez V. and Lyons M. (1995) Interrater reliability of the Glasgow Coma Scale. *Journal of Neuroscience Nursing*, 27(5): 283–286.

Malkmus M. and Stenderup K. (1974) http://www.neuroskills.com/~cns/tbi/rancho.html

Chapter 8

Neurological observations (II): eyes

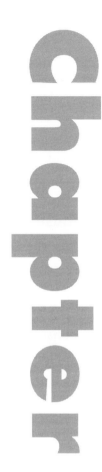

- Introduction
- The basic neurology of the human eye
- Visual disturbance
- Basic eye observations
- Advanced visual neurobiology
- Advanced eye observations
- Key points

Introduction

It has been said that the eyes are the window on the soul. However, for medical purposes, it would be more accurate to say that the eyes are the window on the brain. This is because observation of the eyes gives so many clues about pathological changes taking place within the brain. This should not be surprising since the light-sensitive retina at the back of the eye is the only part of the nervous system visible from the outside world.

The basic neurology of the human eye

This is a simplified account of the complex nervous system that consists of both motor and sensory nerves and their control areas of the brain that serve the eye.

The sensory system (vision)

The sensory nerve component is the visual pathway extending from the retina posteriorly into the brain. Light passes through the **pupil** at the front of the eye onto the **retina** at the back (Figure 8.1). The majority of light falls on that part of the retina that lies directly opposite the pupil: the **macula**, the central part of which is the **fovea**. The fovea has the greatest concentration of daylight-sensitive cells, the **cones**. The straight line from the pupil to the retina is known as the **visual axis**. Cones produce nerve impulses in response to daylight and colour, unlike the other type of light-sensitive cells, the **rods**, which create impulses in response to low light levels and black and white stimuli. Just off-centre to the macula, i.e. a little divergent from the visual axis, is the **optic disc** (Figure 8.2), the area where the retina attaches to the **optic nerve** (Figure 8.1). This nerve is the sensory pathway of vision from the eye: the second cranial nerve (cranial nerve II), which passes posteriorly through the rear of the orbit into the brain.

The left and right optic nerves converge at the **optic chiasma** (Figure 8.3). By the definition of the word nerve (i.e. pathways *outside* the brain and cord), the visual pathways are called the optic nerves *only* from the retina to the chiasma.

The optic chiasma is the point where 50% of the fibres cross to the opposite side (cross-over = **decussation**) (Figure 8.3). The **temporal** (outer) half of each retina generates impulses that remain ipsilateral (=

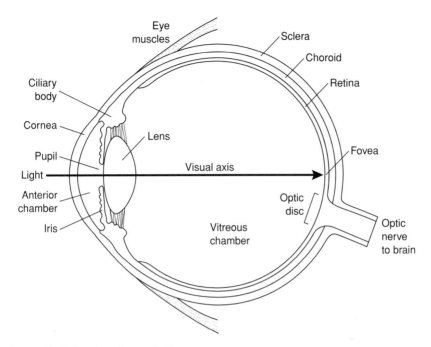

Figure 8.1 Section through the eye.

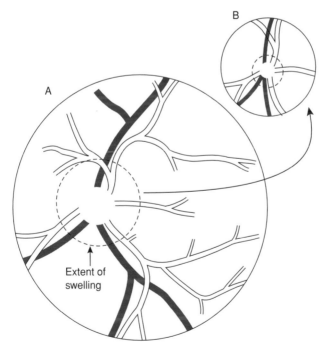

Figure 8.2 View of the retina through an ophthalmoscope. A, papilloedema, with the extent of the optic disc swelling indicated; B, a normal optic disc.

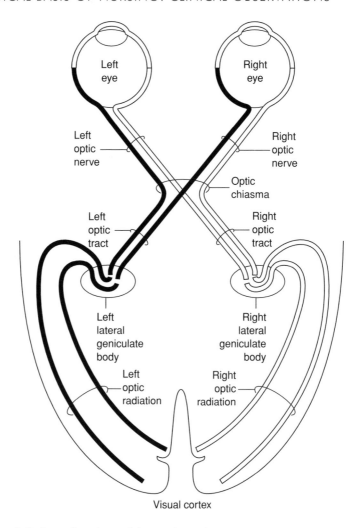

FIGURE 8.3 Superior view of the optic pathways.

on the same side) through the chiasma, whereas the **nasal** (inner) half of each retina generates impulses that decussate, i.e. cross to the opposite side in the chiasma. The result is that each half of the brain, both left and right, receives visual impulses from the temporal retina of the same side but impulses from the nasal retina of the opposite side. But despite this, the brain interprets these signals as a normal complete visual image.

From the chiasma backwards to the thalamus the pathways are *inside* the brain and are therefore called the **optic tracts** (Figure 8.3). After the thalamus, the main pathways continue posteriorly as the **optic radiations**, and these terminate at the back of the brain in the **visual**

cortex within part of the **cerebrum** called the **occipital lobe** (Figure 8.3). Here, the visual stimulus becomes conscious, i.e. we actually see with the rear of the brain, *not* the eye. The retina converts light to nerve impulses that pass through these pathways subconsciously until they reach the visual cortex, at which point we become aware of them. Of course, all these pathways are crucial in the delivery of the impulses to the visual cortex, which is why **blindness** can occur from a disorder at any point along this pathway. The area of vision we see before us constitutes the **visual fields**, the centre of which falls on the visual axis and is the point of our gaze. Nothing that exists outside the periphery of the visual fields can be seen without turning our eyes and head (re-centring our gaze).

The motor system (movements inside and outside the eye)

The motor supply to the eye operates the three muscular aspects of vision: (1) muscle movements of the *whole* eye within the **orbit** (the socket); (2) the movement of the **iris** governing pupil size; and (3) the movement of the **lens** for the purpose of accommodation (focusing on objects at differing distances from the eye).

1 Movement of the whole eye is achieved by the six *striated* muscles *outside* each eye but *within* the orbits. These muscles are controlled by **cranial nerve III**, the **oculomotor** nerve, part of which innervates four of the orbital muscles on both sides; **cranial nerve IV**, the **trochlear** nerve, which innervates one orbital muscle on each side (the **superior oblique**); and **cranial nerve VI**, the **abducens** nerve, which innervates one other orbital muscle on each side (the **lateral rectus**) (Figure 8.4). Cranial nerves are so-called because they come directly from the brain (i.e. *not* via the cord), with cranial nerves III, IV and VI arising in nuclei within the **brain stem**; III and IV in the **midbrain;** and VI in the **pons**. They operate a **reciprocal innervation** of the muscles, i.e. contracting one muscle while relaxing the muscle that moves in the opposite direction. This allows the eyes to both move in one direction at a time, i.e. the eye muscles are **yoked**, which means that their movements are tied together. Although this brain stem function is automatic, it can also occur at a conscious level from the cerebrum (see Chapter 7). In addition, the oculomotor nerve also operates striated muscle that elevates the upper lid.

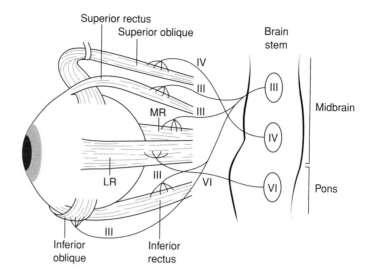

FIGURE 8.4 The external (skeletal) eye muscles and their innervation from the brain stem nuclei of the cranial nerves III, IV and VI. LR, lateral rectus muscle; MR, medial rectus muscle.

2 Pupil size is a function of *smooth* muscle activity *inside* the eye. Pupils respond to light stimuli automatically; the smooth muscle is operated by the **autonomic nervous system (ANS)**, which has both **sympathetic** and **parasympathetic** components. **Pupil constriction** is caused by the *parasympathetic* component of the oculomotor nerve, which innervates the iris **sphincter** muscles in response to bright light. In low light the *sympathetic* controls the iris **radial dilator** muscles and opens the pupil, i.e. **pupil dilatation**. The sympathetic supply to the smooth muscle of the iris comes from the upper thoracic spinal cord (T1 to T3, i.e. first to third thoracic vertebral level), part of the **sympathetic outflow** (Figure 8.5). Thus, the sympathetic is a *spinal* outflow (cord and spinal nerves) whilst the parasympathetic is a *cranial* outflow (medulla and cranial nerve III); a point of importance when considering pupil observations as part of head injury care.

3 The *parasympathetic* component of the oculomotor nerve (cranial nerve III) also controls **accommodation**. This is the process of stretching or relaxing the suspensory smooth muscles that control the shape of the lens for the purpose of focusing on objects that are different distances from the eye. The **near point** is the closest an object can get to the eye and remain in focus, and the eye should be able to focus on an object from this point to infinity.

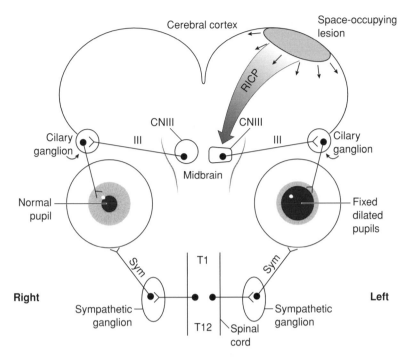

Figure 8.5 Pupil size innervation in normal conditions (right) and in head injury (left). The parasympathetic supply that constricts the pupil comes via the third cranial nerve (III) from the cranial nerve III nuclei (CNIII) in the midbrain. They reach the pupil via the ciliary ganglion. The sympathetic (sym) supply to the eye that dilates the pupil comes from the thoracic spinal cord; the sympathetic emerges from the cord between vertebrae T1 and T12 via the sympathetic ganglion. Raised intracranial pressure (RICP) comes from a space-occupying lesion and compresses the nucleus on the same side causing ipsilateral fixed dilated pupil.

Visual disturbance

Opacity of the lens, called a **cataract**, will prevent light from entering the posterior chamber of the eye. The lens is normally made from clear cells to allow light through, but they are unable to receive a direct blood supply since blood entering the lens would mean that we would see the world through a volume of blood, giving us a permanent red view of the world. This would obviously be disadvantageous for us as well as unpleasant, so these cells must acquire their nutrients and oxygen via a pass along system. In this system, the cells at the edges collect what is needed from the blood and pass it, cell by cell, to all the others in the lens. Waste products flow in the opposite direction. Failure of this transport mechanism, as can occur in old age or exposure to prolonged radiation from the sun, leads to the milky opacity seen in cataracts. This is an observable sign that the cells are not getting adequate nutrients or oxygen and are dying. Cataracts are still a common cause of blindness, especially in developing countries, despite the fact that the relatively simple operation of cataract removal can restore sight quickly.

Glaucoma is a disturbance of vision with acute eye pain that is caused by raised intraoccular pressure, i.e. the fluid inside the front of the eye builds up in volume and then stretches the front of the eye. Patients complain not only of the severe pain but of seeing distorted images surrounded by a halo. The urgent treatment is to administer drops to constrict the pupil (see p. 177) to improve drainage of the front chamber of the eye. Long-term treatment may require surgery to remove a segment of the iris (a partial **iridectomy**), creating a **keyhole** pupil, which nurses may observe in patients with a history of the disease.

Damage or death of cells in the retina, as may occur from looking directly at the sun, or detachment of the retina from the inner wall of the eye can all impair vision. Anything that interrupts the function of the optic nerve, like pressure from a tumour or injury, will block impulses from the retina from reaching the brain. Inside the brain, similar tumour growths, bleeding (as in strokes) or trauma from head injuries can disrupt the pathways from the chiasma to the thalamus or on to the visual cortex of the occipital lobe. The visual cortex itself can be affected by intracranial bleeds, infarcts or direct injury causing trauma to the cells that interpret what we see. It seems odd that loss of vision can be the result of a blow to the back of the head. Some blind patients report only a partial visual loss, which could be a reduction in the ability to see light across the entire visual field, or it may be a narrowing of the field itself. Defects of the visual fields can be detected on examination or reported by the patient. **Tunnel vision** is one such defect, where the peripheral aspects of the fields are gradually or suddenly lost; the patient only sees what is on or close to the visual axis.

Basic eye observations

Pupil size and reaction to light

The normal average pupillary size is about 3.5 mm, with a range from 2 to 6 mm diameter. A light shone into one eye should cause a fast constriction of the pupils in both eyes, a **direct reaction** in the pupil to which the light was applied and a **consensual reaction** in the opposite pupil. The opposite pupil reacts because some branches of the neuronal connections in the brain stem decussate, whereas others remain ipsilateral (Figure 8.6). The pupil size is partly governed by a **pupillary reflex**, an autonomic motor response to the sensory stimulus of light intensity falling on the retina. As noted above (p. 172), the reflex action to bright light has a sensory input from the retina, the optic nerve (cranial nerve II); a motor output to the pupillary muscles of the iris, the parasympathetic oculomotor nerve (cranial nerve III); and brain stem relay areas (Figure 8.6). Pupil size is also partly governed by optical needs, the pupil will constrict as part of the mechanism for regulating depth of focus, and under these circumstances the constriction is independent of light intensity (Hickey 1997).

Abnormal pupils

Abnormal pupils are an important nursing observation and require careful interpretation and sometimes urgent intervention. Blindness in one eye due to causes involving the front of the eye, the retina or the optic nerve will mean the loss of the sensory component of the light pupillary reflex. Light shone in the blind eye will not affect either pupil size, but light will cause pupillary constriction in *both* eyes if it is shone in the good eye (provided the oculomotor nerve is functioning). Blindness caused by problems *inside* the brain are beyond the pupillary reflex and the pupils should therefore still react to light.

  Pinpoint pupils (**miotic pupils**) (Figure 8.7) is where pupillary size is at its minimum, i.e. the pupils are just visible at 1 mm or less in diameter, and are unlikely to constrict further to light. **Opiate drugs**, such as heroin, in large doses can cause this, and pinpoint pupils is a sign used to observe for opiate abuse. Alternatively, it may be caused by anything that obstructs the sympathetic supply to the eye, thus allowing the parasympathetic full control, e.g. spinal lesions with cervical nerve damage, causing **Horner's pupil** (see p. 186 and Figure 8.7). Pinpoint pupils may also be a feature of direct orbital trauma (identified by other signs of orbital injury, like bruising). Small pupils (i.e. smaller than 3 mm) are naturally going to occur in bright light, and should be capable of further constriction if the light gets brighter. Abnormal small pupils could be the result of any of the conditions identified under pinpoint pupils, but to a lesser degree. In addition, if the small pupils

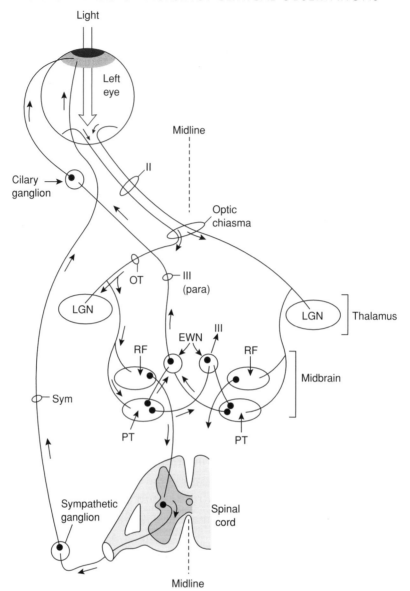

FIGURE 8.6 Diagram showing detail of the pathways involved in establishing pupil size in response to light. Light enters the eye and impulses return to the brain from the retina via the optic nerve (II, cranial nerve II). Medial retinal impulses cross the midline at the optic chiasma; lateral retinal impulses do not cross. Impulses then pass to the lateral geniculate nucleus (LGN) via the optic tracts (OT). Some impulses are redirected to the reticular formation (RF) and the pretectum (PT). From the pretectum the impulses pass to the Edinger–Westphal nucleus (EWN), which is part of the cranial nerve III (III, oculomotor nerve) nucleus. This nerve provides parasympathetic (para) innervation to the pupil via the ciliary ganglion to cause constriction in bright light. From the reticular formation pathways descend the spinal cord to the sympathetic output of the thoracic cord. From here the pupil is supplied with sympathetic (Sym) fibres that dilate the pupil in dull light. Only the left side is shown.

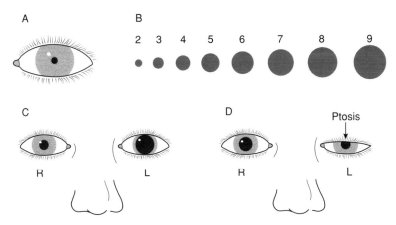

FIGURE 8.7 Pupil sizes. A, pinpoint pupils; B, various sizes from 2 to 9 mm; C, unilateral fixed dilated pupil on the left seen in oculomotor nerve compression or damage due to raised intracranial pressure; D, Horner's syndrome, with right dilated pupil and left ptosis.

are bilateral and respond to light, they could also be found in comas caused by a number of abnormal metabolic conditions (e.g. diabetic ketoacidosis or coma due to imbalance of blood electrolytes), or they could be due to bilateral injury to the thalamus or hypothalamus (**bilateral diencephalic damage**). Small irregular pupils that do *not* react to light but do constrict on accommodation of close objects are called **Argyll Robertson** pupils, and have long been associated with **syphilis** (a sexually transmitted infection involving the brain), but can also be a feature of other brain stem disorders. Small or pinpoint pupils can result from the use of miotic drugs, such as pilocarpine or physostigmine, as a treatment for glaucoma (see p. 174).

Normal average-sized pupils that, however, are *not* reacting to light indicate a failure of both components of the autonomic nervous system and may be a feature of midbrain injury from **infarction** (a sudden loss of blood supply leading to an area of dead or dying tissue) or **herniation** (part of the brain forced out of position, usually downwards).

Dilation of the pupils (or **mydriasis**, 6–8 mm diameter) occurs normally in low light conditions, but the pupils will constrict again on exposure to light (Figure 8.7). Pupil dilation can also be caused by high-dosage **amphetamines** (nervous system stimulants) or **glutethimide** (a sedative), or by the use of a **mydriatic** or **cycloplegic** drugs for eye examination purposes. These drugs (e.g. tropicamide, cyclopentolate and homatropine) dilate the pupil by blocking the parasympathetic and thus increasing the sympathetic balance to the eye. Large pupils may also be due to direct orbital injuries (as with small pupils) if the trauma causes pressure on the third cranial nerve with concurrent loss of pupillary constriction.

Chapter 7 identified the abnormal changes in pupil size and reaction to light as a focal sign of raised intracranial pressure (RICP), but they could be due to other intracranial disorders. In head injury, these changes are initially a dilated pupil that is *unilateral* (on one side), *ipsilateral* (the same side as the injury) and *fixed* (no response to light). Later (and this could be anything from minutes to hours), the fixed dilated pupil becomes *bilateral* (both sides). The time taken for the progression from unilateral to bilateral is dependent on the rate of increase in the SOL that is causing the increased pressure, e.g. the extradural haematoma, which progresses much faster than the subdural haematoma in head injuries (see Chapter 7). The observation made is twofold; first identification of the size of the pupil on both sides so that equality of the left pupil with the right can be assessed, and second the pupil's reaction to light. Pupils that are widely dilated (9 mm or more in diameter) and fixed (not reacting to light) is a very serious observation suggesting intracranial bleeding after head injury, or some other SOL, such as a brain tumour or cerebral oedema and must be reported and acted upon urgently. Raised intracranial pressure (RICP) from the developing SOL causes failure of the brain stem areas controlling pupil constriction or compression of the oculomotor nerve. This is often unilateral at first, leading to bilateral as the RICP increases, causing compression down onto the brain stem. Continued compression of the brain stem as the SOL gets larger will result in **coning**, a herniation of parts of the brain, including the medulla, downwards into the foramen magnum at the base of the skull. As the cardiac and respiratory centres are there, they will be compressed and both the heart and the lungs will stop functioning, with little chance of resuscitation. Fixed, bilateral dilated pupils are also seen in the terminal stages of many conditions including **cerebral ischaemia** (loss of blood supply to the brain) and severe **cerebral anoxia** (loss of oxygen); and indeed it is also the state seen after death has occurred. Neuroscience nurses may need a more advanced text on various pupil responses, e.g. Hickey (1997).

Advanced visual neurobiology

Sensory pathways

The optic tracts link the chiasma with parts of the thalamus (see Chapter

7, p. 143) known as the **lateral geniculate nucleus (LGN)**. About 10% of the visual stimulus passing along this optic tract connects with part of the **midbrain,** the superior colliculus (Figure 8.8). This area responds to retinal impulses by operating the muscles that are keeping the eye and head in a position to retain the viewed image on the fovea. It is therefore responsible for maintaining the eye's *gaze* on a subject, especially if that subject is moving. The superior colliculus is linked to the three cranial nerves operating the orbital muscles that move the

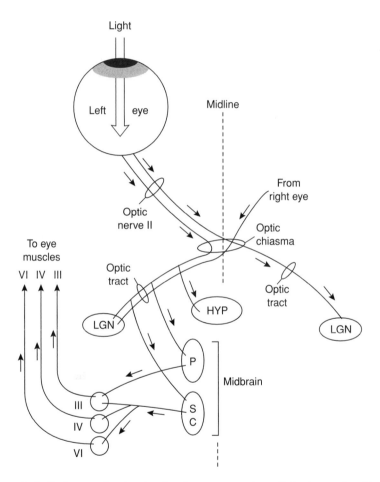

FIGURE 8.8 Pathways in the brain that respond to light intensity. Nerve impulses passing down the optic nerve not only go to the lateral geniculate nucleus (LGN, on the visual pathway), but some pass to the hypothalamus (HYP), which governs the sleep–wake cycle in response to light intensity. Some also pass to the pretectum (P), which helps to control pupil size, and some go to the superior colliculus (SC), which aids in eye movements via the cranial nerves III, IV and VI. Only the left side is shown.

eye (see p. 182). These muscles are attached to the external surface of the eyeball. Gaze is a vital requirement for hunting and survival, and in lower vertebrates the superior colliculus is the main area to which *all* the retinal output goes. The fact that only 10% of the pathway goes there in humans suggests that it may be less important for us, although 10% of *human* retinal output is roughly the equivalent to the *entire* retinal output of a cat (Bear *et al.* 1996). Another area of the midbrain that receives light-induced impulses is the **pretectum**, the relay nucleus that has partial control over pupil size and some eye movements in response to light intensity. The pretectum is an intermediary link between the incoming sensory impulses from the retina and the outgoing motor impulses of the parasympathetic third cranial nerve (see p. 179). A final area that receives light-induced impulses from the optic tracts is the **hypothalamus** (Figure 8.8). Here the sleep–wake cycle is controlled by the light intensity falling on the retina and transmitted as impulses to the hypothalamus via the optic tracts. This cycle determines when the brain will sleep (in response to low light) and when it will awake (in response to greater light).

The retina causes impulses to travel along the optic nerve (sensory) to the pretectum, then onto the **Edinger–Westphal nucleus**, which is part of **the third cranial nerve nucleus** in the midbrain (Figures 8.6 and 8.8). The Edinger–Westphal nucleus is the pupillary control centre and origin of the *parasympathetic* component of the oculomotor nerve. From here, the oculomotor nerve passes to the orbit, where a **synapse** occurs with the cell body of the second neurones, called the **ciliary ganglion**, before the nerve entering the iris. Second, neurones of the oculomotor nerve also pass from the ciliary ganglion into the **ciliary body** inside the eye, where they control suspensory *smooth* muscles that pull on the lens. The first neurones of the *sympathetic* outflow pass down the upper thoracic spinal nerves into the **sympathetic trunk** on each side of the spine and then pass up the trunk to synapse with the **superior cervical ganglion**, the cell body of the second neurones. From here the second neurones pass up towards the head and follow the arterial pathway into the eyes.

Motor system and eye movements

Eye movements are essential to allow the subject of visual interest to remain on the fovea when it is stationary (**gaze holding**) or moving (**gaze shifting**) and also to respond quickly to new visual stimuli entering the visual fields. A rapid eye movement (or sudden attention change) in order to bring a new or peripheral object onto the fovea is called a **saccade**. Saccades are the fastest specialised form of *gaze shift* and can be vertical, horizontal or a combination of these. Vertical saccades are controlled by an area at the highest point of the midbrain, close to the thalamus, from where connections pass to the oculomotor and trochlear nuclei. Horizontal saccades are commanded from lower in the brain stem, close to the pons (Figure 8.9). Bilateral lesions in either of these command areas, as may be possible in brain stem ischaemia or bleeds, can result in a loss of the corresponding saccade. Other gaze shifts

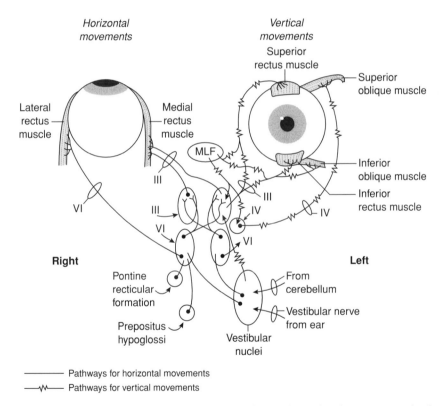

FIGURE 8.9 Control of eye movements. The right side shows control of horizontal movements. Input to the cranial nerve VI nucleus is from the pontine reticular formation, the vestibular nuclei and the prepositus hypoglossi. The cranial nerve VI nucleus connects to the cranial nerve III nucleus on both sides. The left side shows control of vertical movements. Input to the cranial nerve III nucleus is from the cerebellum and vestibular nerve via the vestibular nuclei and from the medial longitudinal fasciculus (MLF), which also has direct output to the superior and inferior rectus muscles.

include **smooth pursuit** (retains the image of a moving object on the fovea) and **vergence** (the eyes move in opposing directions to retain the image simultaneously on both foveae). These are conscious motor activities and are therefore controlled by specific areas of the cerebral cortex (Figure 8.10). Since they are in response to visual sensory stimuli, neuronal connections occur between the sensory visual cortex in the occipital lobe and the various ophthalmic motor centres of the parietal and frontal lobes. From these centres motor pathways descend through the basal ganglia and via the superior colliculus, the gaze control centre, with output to the cranial nerve nuclei in the brain stem that govern eye muscle movement. In general, nuclei in the midbrain (cranial nerves III and IV) control vertical gaze, whereas the nucleus in the pons (cranial nerve VI) controls horizontal gaze.

Advanced eye observations

Abnormal eye movements

Nurses may note abnormalities of both gaze holding and gaze shift in conscious patients (but to a much lesser extent in an unconscious patient

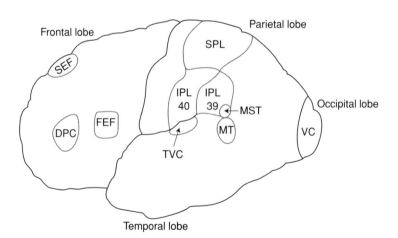

FIGURE 8.10 Areas of the cerebral cortex involved in eye movement control. DPC, dorsolateral prefrontal cortex (area 46); FEF, frontal eye fields (parts of areas 4, 6, 8, 9); IPL inferior parietal lobe (areas 39, 40); MST, medial superior temporal visual area (parts of areas 19, 37, 39); MT, mid-temporal visual areas (parts of areas 19, 37); SEF, supplementary eye fields (part of area 6); SPL superior parietal lobe (areas 5, 7); TVC, temporal vestibular cortex (parts of areas 41, 42); VC, visual cortex (area 17).

who is unable to co-operate). Abnormal gaze holding can be seen in unilateral paralysis of each of the cranial nerves that control eye muscles, and these present with the characteristic symptom of the two eyes no longer functioning together (Figure 8.11). **Diagonal diplopia** (diplopia = double vision) is seen in unilateral **cranial nerve III palsy** (paralysis of one oculomotor nerve), where the eye *on the affected side* looks 'down and out' with ptosis (see p. 186) and pupil dilatation, while the other eye appears normal. Unilateral **cranial nerve IV palsy** results in a **vertical diplopia**, as the eye on the affected side becomes unable to

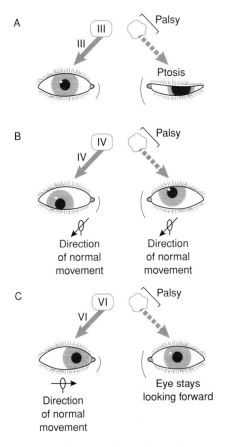

FIGURE 8.11 Disturbance of eye positions in various cranial nerve palsy. A, cranial nerve III causes the 'down and out' appearance of the affected eye with dilated pupil and ptosis of the lid; B, cranial nerve IV palsy causes the affected eye to have limited ability to look down when it is adducted (moved towards the nose); C, cranial nerve VI palsy causes the inability to abduct (move towards the ear) the affected eye when both eyes are commanded to look in that direction.

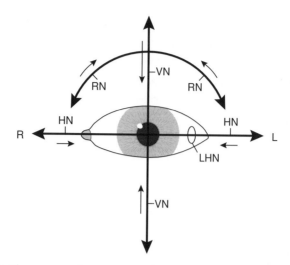

FIGURE 8.12 The range of movements in nystagmus. Nystagmus has a slow movement phase (short, thin arrow) and a rapid return phase (long, thick arrow). The rapid phase is the direction given for the nystagmus (HN), rotary nystagmus (RN) or a mix of these in either left, right, up or down directions.

look down when adducted (brought towards the nose). Unilateral **cranial nerve VI palsy** causes **horizontal diplopia,** as the affected eye cannot be abducted (moved outwards) (Figure 8.11).

Abnormal *gaze shift* may be seen when the patient is asked to follow the examiner's finger through a range of up, down, left and right movements. **Nystagmus** describes the involuntary rhythmic oscillations of the eyeball, a rapid back and forth movement that the patient has no control over (Figure 8.12). Nystagmus may occur in the horizontal, vertical, mixed or rotary directions. Two types of nystagmus have been identified: the more common *jerky* form, in which movements in one direction are faster (rapid saccade) than in the other direction, or the *pendular* form, in which the movements in both directions are equal in speed. Nystagmus can be artificially induced in normal individuals by putting cold water into an ear, a procedure called a **cold caloric** test. It causes **vestibular** (= balance or equilibrium) stimulation by chilling the fluid within **the lateral semicircular canal,** part of the **labyrinth** (= cavity) of the inner ear, and thus creating convection currents in this fluid. This tests the function of the pathway passing from the semicircular canals of the inner ear (the vestibular branch of cranial nerve VIII) to the brain stem and **cerebellum,** then on to the cranial nerve nuclei controlling eye movements (see p. 171). The cerebellum controls balance (in response to semicircular canal activity) and both the speed and the co-ordination of eye saccades. **Labyrinthine vestibular nystagmus**, a rotary jerky form, may be caused by diseases of the inner ear. Other jerky forms can be caused by brain stem or cerebellar diseases, or as the result of barbiturate overdose. Pendular nystagmus is usually a feature of **intraocular disease**, i.e. disorders of the retina or fluid pressures inside the eye. For a more advanced text on eye movements see Downey and Leigh (1998).

Papilloedema

Papilloedema is swelling of the optic disc due to oedema. Using an **ophthalmoscope** the retina is viewed (known as a **funduscopic examination** since the **fundus**, or deepest part of the eye where the retina lies, will be seen), and the retinal blood vessels can been identified (Figure 8.2). These vessels spread out to all parts of the retina from a single point, the optic disc, just off centre from the macula. The blood vessels are the **retinal arteries and veins**, the blood supply to this light-sensitive layer, and they follow the optic nerve pathway between the brain and the eye. The veins are some 30% larger than the arteries, but like everywhere else, the retinal arteries carry blood at greater pressure than the veins. Papilloedema is usually caused by raised intracranial pressure (RICP, see Chapter 7). This is because the meninges surrounding the brain are continuous along the optic nerve to the optic disc, and any RICP will exist along the optic nerve and onto the disc itself. When pressure is applied to the blood vessels from RICP the veins will tend to be occluded before the arteries (i.e. at an early stage of RICP). This means that blood passing along the vessels enters the retina easier via the arteries than it can leave via the veins. The RICP together with some venous congestion causes excess tissue fluid to accumulate, called oedema, at the point around the vessel entry, the optic disc. This obscures the normally obvious disc margins; they become distorted and swollen, with the disc becoming a reddish colour, i.e. visual proof of the existence of RICP. This becomes a very important visual check for RICP (remember the statement at the start about the retina being the only part of the nervous system visible from the outside world). It is not only carried out as part of the neurological examination of the patient but is usually also done to exclude the existence of RICP before a **lumbar puncture** (LP). A lumbar puncture is the introduction of a needle into the spinal canal below the level of **lumbar vertebra 2 (L2)** in order to obtain a sample of **cerebrospinal fluid (CSF)**. If RICP was present during a lumbar puncture, the sudden decompression of the cord by removing CSF could cause coning (see p. 161).

Ptosis

The elevation of the upper eyelid is a function of the oculomotor nerve (see p. 171) and incomplete opening of the upper lid is a condition called ptosis (or lid lag). It can be seen by observing the narrowed **palpebral fissure**, i.e. the gap between the upper and lower lids, when the patient is asked to open the eyes. Ptosis may be unilateral or bilateral, and may be the result of oculomotor nerve or brain stem injury or compression, as in raised intracranial pressure. In could be part of several neurological disorders, e.g. **Horner's syndrome**, where ptosis, constricted pupils and dry facial skin indicate the presence of a spinal cord lesion (syndrome = a collection of symptoms that tend to be present together) (Figure 8.7). Some drugs, e.g. the **benzodiazepines**, such as Valium, may cause ptosis when given in sufficient dosage to induce sedation before minor surgical procedures.

Key points

- The optic nerve (cranial nerve II) is the sensory nerve of vision from the eye. It passes posteriorly into the brain.
- The left and right optic nerves converge at the optic chiasma.
- The optic tracts link the chiasma with the lateral geniculate nucleus (LGN), part of the thalamus.
- Ten per cent of the visual stimulus passing along this optic tract connects with the superior colliculus, part of the midbrain. This area operates the muscles that keep the eye fixed on an image, maintaining the gaze.
- The pretectum in the midbrain receives retinal impulses and has partial control over pupil size and some eye movements in response to light intensity.
- Posteriorly to the LGN, the optic radiations pass to the visual cortex, part of the occipital lobe of the cerebrum.
- Cranial nerve III (oculomotor) innervates four of the orbital muscles, cranial nerve IV (trochlear) innervates the superior oblique muscle, and cranial nerve VI (abducens) innervates the lateral rectus muscle.

- The third cranial nerve nucleus in the medulla contains the Edinger–Westphal area, the pupillary constriction centre and origin of the parasympathetic component of the oculomotor nerve.
- The sympathetic supply to the iris comes from the upper thoracic spinal cord (T1 to T3), part of the sympathetic outflow, and causes pupillary dilatation.
- The pupil size is partly due to a pupillary reflex, an autonomic motor response to the sensory stimulus of light intensity falling on the retina, and partly due to optical adjustments required for depth of focus.
- Miotic pupils are pinpoint, and mydriatic pupils are dilated. Miotic and mydriatic drugs can be used to close and open the pupils respectively.
- Unilateral, followed by bilateral widely dilated and fixed pupils may be due to intracranial bleeding after a head injury and must be reported urgently.
- A rapid eye movement or sudden attention change is called a saccade.
- Nystagmus is the rapid involuntary rhythmic back and forth movement (fast saccades) of the eyeball and may be due to vestibular (balance) disorder, intraoccular diseases or barbiturate overdose.
- Diplopia is double vision.
- Papilloedema is swelling of the optic disc and is visual proof of the existence of RICP.
- Incomplete opening of the upper lid is a condition called ptosis (or lid lag).

References

Bear M., Connors B. and Paradiso M. (1996) *Neuroscience, Exploring the Brain*. Williams and Wilkins, Baltimore.

Downey D. and Leigh R. (1998) Eye movements: Pathophysiology, examination and clinical importance. *Journal of Neuroscience Nursing*, 30(1): 15–24.

Hickey J. V. (1997) *The Clinical Practice of Neurological and Neurosurgical Nursing*, 4th edn. Lippincott, Philadelphia.

Chapter 9

Neurological observations (III): movement

- Introduction
- The neurology of human movement
- Movement observations
- Movement losses
- Movement excesses
- The immobile patient
- Key points

Introduction

The ability to move is fundamental to our existence and survival. It therefore becomes life threatening when movement is disturbed by disease or injury, requiring a great deal of nursing care.

We are not born with full movement; indeed the human newborn is extremely limited in what movement it can make. Most movements achieved by adult age are learnt throughout childhood; often after bitter trial and error. This learning process does not involve gaining extra neurones; we are born with about twenty billion neurones and gradually lose them through life. Learning is still somewhat of a mystery, but it seems that it involves gaining both neuronal connections, called synapses, and specific chemical receptors at those synapses. The normal child will gain the usual movement abilities, such as walking and talking, but specific movement skills, like playing the piano, require additional learning involving considerable practice. Despite how much we take it for granted, movement, it seems, does not come easy. This is partly due to the complexity of the motor system, which has far more to do than just control muscles.

The neurology of human movement

This simplified version of motor activity introduces the concepts of muscle movement in relation to balance and posture, muscle tone, co-ordination and smoothing out of muscle activity, special skills like synergy (see p. 201) and the importance of sensory feedback.

We do have conscious control over the obvious movements; we can decide when to walk, to grasp an object, and so on. There are, however, many thousands of subconscious (or automatic) muscle changes and neuronal activities going on continuously, many of which make the conscious movements possible.

Conscious muscle control begins with the **primary motor cortex** within the frontal lobe of the cerebrum. Cells here are the start of the pyramidal system which initiates the contraction of the skeletal muscle that moves the body (Figure 9.1). The **pyramidal system** is so named because it forms a pyramid shape as it passes down through the brain. Consciousness suggests that each movement is purposefully thought about, but in reality we move *without* thinking. Most movements are pre-programmed and require little if any thought. Pre-programming of movement is the essence of the learning process and has been discussed earlier (p. 190). This is seen in the pianist who plays a

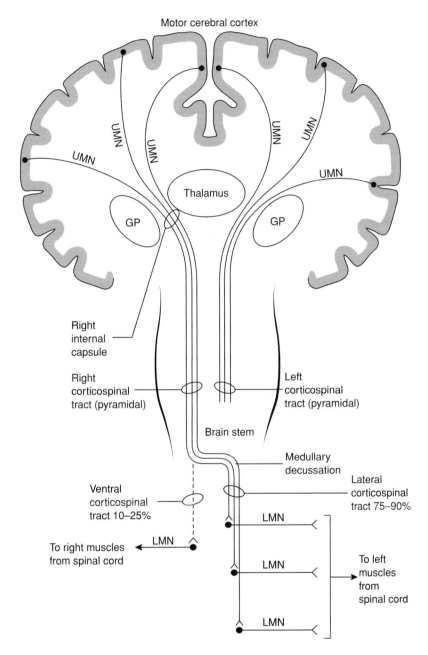

FIGURE 9.1 The pyramidal tracts. The corticospinal (known as pyramidal) tracts begin with widely distributed neuronal cell bodies within the motor cortex (three shown) on both sides. The collected pathway passes between the globus pallidus (GP) and the thalamus at the internal capsule. The fibres (70–90%) cross (decussate) to the opposite side (contralateral) in the medulla to form the lateral corticospinal tract; 10–25% remain on the same side (ipsilateral) to form the ventral corticospinal tract. LMN, lower motor neurone; UMN, upper motor neurone.

Beethoven sonata effortlessly, the finger movements being pre-programmed by years of practice. The conscious aspect involves the ability to initiate the movement in response to sensory stimuli, to be aware of the movement as it happens and to modify the motor response according to sensory feedback. The muscle co-ordination, extent and smoothness of contraction, repetition of muscle action (as in running) and other features of movement are controlled at a subconscious level by the **extra-pyramidal** system (extra = outside, i.e. a system outside the pyramidal system functioning at an automatic level; see p. 196).

The parietal association cortex and motor planning

Voluntary movement is usually in response to sensory stimuli, and the site for the integration of the sensory stimuli is the **parietal association cortex** in the **posterior parietal lobe** of the cerebrum (Figure 9.2). Input to this area comes from the visual cortex (vision), the auditory cortex (hearing) and the somatic sensory cortex (touch). Output from this centre is to two motor areas in the frontal lobes, the **premotor cortex** and the **supplementary motor area** (SMA). The parietal association cortex is thought to work by establishing the *spatial co-ordinates* of objects, i.e. the position of the object in space, in the

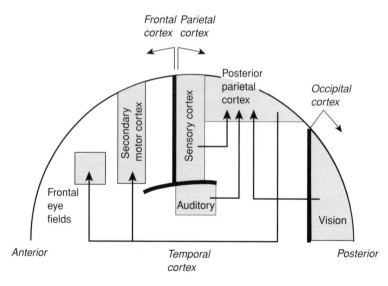

FIGURE 9.2 A schematic diagram of the parietal association cortex showing inputs from the somatosensory, auditory and visual areas, and outputs to the secondary motor cortex and frontal eye fields.

environment to be moved in some way . Once this information is sent to the frontal lobe, the premotor cortex works out the voluntary muscle movements required to interact with any object *seen* by the person, i.e. in response to the visual stimuli from the parietal association cortex. At the same time, the supplementary motor area provides a plan of voluntary muscle movements required for the interaction with an object *touched*, i.e. mainly in response to somatic (= body) stimuli organised by the parietal association cortex. Once these frontal lobe motor areas have produced a plan of muscle activity, they forward the data to the primary motor cortex, where muscle function can be initiated (Pinel 1993). Part of the output from the parietal association cortex is also passed to another frontal lobe zone, the **frontal eye fields**, which are important in the control of eye movements during muscle activity intended to interact with a seen object (Figure 9.2).

The pyramidal tract system (Figure 9.1)

The cells of the primary motor cortex are not randomly arranged; rather, they are positioned in a manner that reflects the basic body plan (Figure 9.3). Larger surface areas housing greater cell numbers occur on the

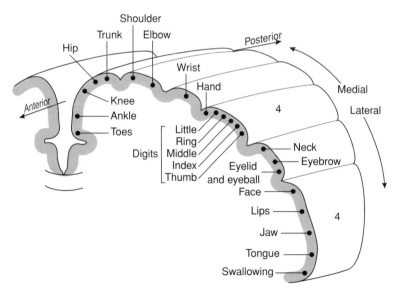

FIGURE 9.3 The left main motor cortex (area 4) showing the layout of the cells according to function (i.e. the muscle sites they control). Notice the large area controlling finger and hand movements compared with the area for feet and toes, which indicates great manual dexterity.

cortex representing those parts where fine intricate muscle movement is required, notably the hands. Pathways descending from the motor cortex, the **pyramidal tracts**, pass through the brain to the brain stem and onward into the cord (Figure 9.1). At the level of the medulla about 75% of these fibres decussate (i.e. cross to the other side) and become contralateral (i.e. from the *opposite* side), whereas the other 25% remain **ipsilateral** (i.e. from the same side). Since both cerebral hemispheres have a motor cortex, there are four pyramidal pathways descending the cord from the brain; two contralateral that have crossed (one from each side, called the **MI** tracts) and two ipsilateral that have not crossed (one on each side, called the **MII** tracts). Neurones occupying these pyramidal tracts are called **upper motor neurones (UMNs)**, i.e. they extend from the brain to the cord within the **central nervous system (CNS)**. The descending MI and MII tracts pass down the spinal cord in specific positions within the **white matter** (Figure 9.4). The fibres enter the anterior **grey matter** of the cord, where they synapse with other neurones at all the spinal levels, i.e. from high in the cervical (neck) region to low in the sacral (pelvic) region.

Lower motor neurones (**LMNs**) are those that begin with the cells in the anterior grey matter of the cord, and the fibres pass via the **anterior root** into the **spinal nerve** to the voluntary skeletal muscles of the body. The LMN is therefore part of the **peripheral nervous system (PNS)**, being a component of the spinal nerves. Therefore, the pyramidal system is two-neuronal, consisting of a UMN and an LMN, from motor cortex to muscle (Figure 9.1).

The pyramidal system also operates through some of the **cranial nerves** that control muscles of the head, face and neck. The

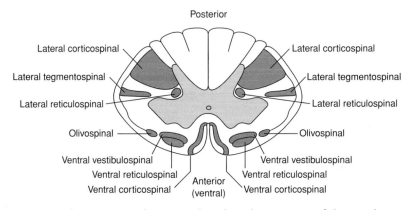

FIGURE 9.4 The motor pathways within the white matter of the cord.

corticobulbar tracts (Figure 9.5) begin as neuronal cell bodies in the head and neck areas (lateral areas) of the motor cortex (hence *cortico*). These UMN fibres pass down to nuclei in the pons and medulla of the brain stem (note: the brain stem is called *bulbar*, i.e. shaped like a bulb). From a nucleus in the *pons*, LMN fibres become components of the **trigeminal nerve** (cranial V) and pass to the muscles of the lower jaw (e.g. for eating). Also from the *pons*, LMN fibres form part of the **facial nerve** (cranial VII) and pass to muscles of the face (e.g. for facial

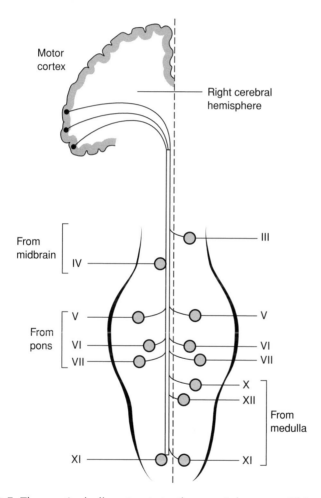

FIGURE 9.5 The corticobulbar tracts to the cranial nerves. This schematic diagram shows motor pathways coming from the head and neck area of the right motor cortex (see Figure 9.3) and passing into the brain stem. The cranial nerve nuclei are indicated, showing their brain stem locations, the corticobulbar input (unilateral or bilateral) which cross the midline. The left hemisphere (not shown) has a mirror image input.

expression). Separate *medullary* nuclei give rise to LMN fibres within the **glossopharyngeal nerve** (cranial IX, to pharyngeal muscles), the **vagus nerve** (cranial X, to muscles of the pharynx, larynx, oesophagus and soft palate) and the **spinal accessory nerve** (cranial XI, to the neck muscles).

The extra-pyramidal system

This system operates skeletal muscle at the subconscious level, i.e. it controls the automatic aspects of voluntary movement. The main areas of the brain involved are (1) parts of the cerebral cortex and the red nucleus; (2) the basal ganglia and parts of the thalamus; (3) parts of the pons and medulla, including all their pathways and feedback circuits (Figure 9.6).

1 Some *primary* cells within the cerebral cortex have fibres that end in the red nucleus within the midbrain, the **corticorubral tract**. In the red nucleus, *secondary* cells give rise to fibres that pass down the cord, forming the **rubrospinal tract**.

2 Several nuclei towards the base of the brain are collectively called the basal ganglia (Figure 9.7). One of these nuclei, the **globus pallidus**, has *primary* cells providing fibres that terminate in some areas of the thalamus. From the thalamus, *secondary* cell fibres feed back to the motor cortex of the cerebrum (part of the basal ganglia motor loop, see p. 198 and Figures 9.6 and 9.9).

3 Areas of the pons and medulla, known as the **reticular formation**, have *secondary* cells with fibres extending down the cord, creating the **reticulospinal tract**.

The basal ganglia and thalamus

The five nuclei of the basal ganglia (Figure 9.7) are responsible for a major influence, both **facilitatory** and **inhibitory**, on movement. Facilitatory promotes movement and inhibitory prevents movement, like an accelerator and a break in a car providing fine control of the vehicle. In particular, these nuclei have a major role in slow, sustained movements and in maintaining **muscle tone** (Figure 9.8). Muscle tone can be described as a state of readiness for contraction; a tension within the muscle which is essential if the muscle is to function instantly when stimulated. Exercise has the effect of increasing muscle tone, as identified by those who attend the gymnasium regularly, and a lack of

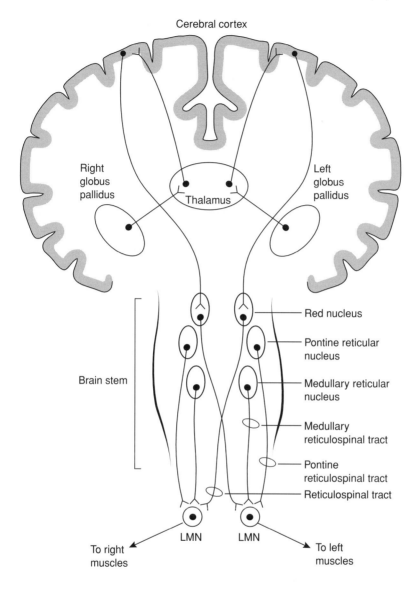

FIGURE 9.6 Some extra-pyramidal tracts. Pathways of the extra-pyramidal system extend from the cerebral cortex to the red nucleus, and from the red nucleus to the contralateral LMN (lower motor neurone) in the cord (a pathway called the rubrospinal tract), from the globus pallidus to the thalamus with feedback pathways to the cortex, from the pontine nucleus to the ipsilateral LMN (called the pontine reticulospinal tract) and from the medullary reticulospinal nucleus to the LMN (called the medullary reticulospinal tract).

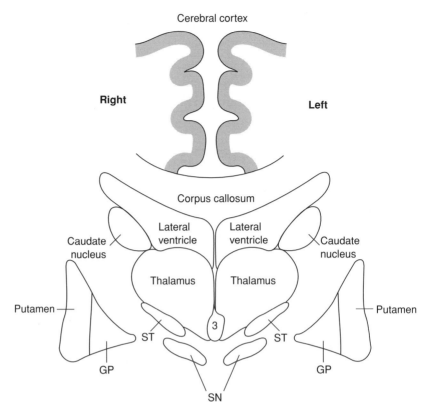

FIGURE 9.7 Areas that make up the basal ganglia. GP, globus pallidus; SN, substantia nigra; ST, subthalamus; 3, third ventricle.

exercise causes a loss of tone. This is one reason why prolonged bed rest is no longer a treatment for patients, for it results in muscle tone loss, i.e. loose, floppy muscles that do not function properly. But this effect is not the only factor since the basal ganglia provide *inhibition* (or *reduction*) of excessive muscle tone, and this is notably a major role of the nucleus called the **substantia nigra** (see p. 209 and Figure 9.7).

A major influence over movement is the **basal ganglia motor loop** (Figure 9.9), in which the globus pallidus *inhibits* part of the thalamus (the **ventral lateral nucleus**, or **VL**) during rest. Activation of the motor cortex of the cerebrum *switches on* another nucleus of the basal ganglia, the **putamen**, part of the **corpus striatum**. This activation of the putamen in turn *inhibits* the globus pallidus, thus removing the inhibition on the thalamus. Free now to act, the thalamus has considerable influence on an area close to the motor cortex, the **supplementary motor area (SMA)**, which in turn focuses the activity

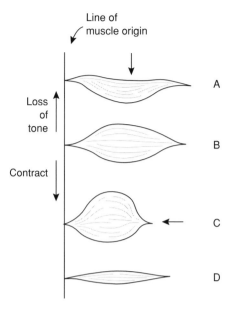

FIGURE 9.8 Muscle tone. A, loss of muscle tone, the muscle is soft loose and floppy, sinking in response to gravity (i.e. after long immobilisation); B, normal muscle tone, the muscle is firm and retains its shape ready for contraction; C, Contraction of the muscle, where the insertion (opposite end to the origin) moves towards the origin (which does not move); D, muscle wasting, where muscle bulk is lost. Excessive muscle tone appears as the opposite of A, i.e. the muscle is tight and stiff and cannot contract normally.

of the main motor cortex. Thus the loop is complete when motor cortex activity switches on the mechanism that focuses that activity.

The cerebellum

The **cerebellum** (Figure 9.10) contributes several aspects of movement, not least of which are **balance** and **posture**. The equilibrium of the body requires the **centre of gravity** (in the mid-lumbar spinal area) to remain within the base, i.e. the floor area occupied by the two feet. Should the centre of gravity drift outside the base, the individual will fall to one side. To prevent this, many minute muscular adjustments are constantly made to keep the body upright inside the base, correcting any defects in posture at the same time. These muscular contractions are co-ordinated by the cerebellum at an unconscious level, but they require *sensory* feedback to tell the cerebellum what the second-by-second state of the body's balance is. This sensory feedback on balance

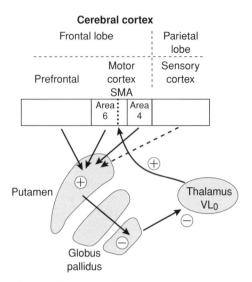

FIGURE 9.9 Basal ganglia motor loop. Input to the putamen comes from the frontal cortex with less input from the parietal sensory cortex. This activates (+) neurones running from the putamen to the globus pallidus, which, in turn, then deactivate (–) neurones linking the globus pallidus with the ventral lateral nucleus of the thalamus (known as VL_0). These globus pallidus neurones prevent (i.e. inhibit, shown as –) any feedback from the VL_0 to the cerebral cortex. However, deactivation from the putamen has removed this inhibition, and the VL_0 then has freedom to feedback to the cortex (+), more precisely the supplemental motor area (SMA) of area 6 of the motor cortex.

(known as **vestibular** stimuli) comes from the semicircular canals of the inner ear, via the **vestibulocochlear nerve** (cranial nerve VIII). Additional sensory information on balance comes from receptors in the joints and muscles; this is sensory feedback called **proprioception** and arrives in the brain stem via the spinal cord. The cerebellum, like the cerebrum, is divided into a left and right **hemisphere**, both of which communicate with the rest of the brain entirely via the brain stem. This is through connections called the **cerebellar peduncles** (ped = foot; the cerebellar feet), and three such peduncles exist: the **superior**, **middle** and **inferior**. The vestibular stimuli from both ears arrive at one of the three cerebellar lobes that occur within each hemisphere, the **flocculonodular lobe**, the area ultimately responsible for balance. Proprioception stimuli arrive at another cerebellar lobe, the **anterior lobe**, where posture can be maintained. The cerebellum's **posterior lobe** receives impulses from the high centres of the cerebrum via the brain stem. These cerebral connections allow the cerebellum to step in

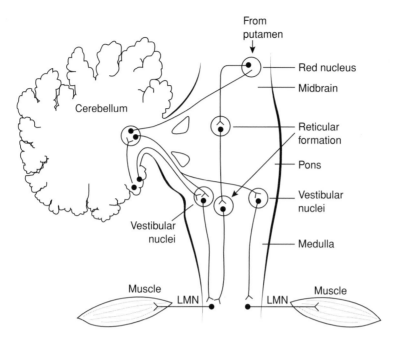

Figure 9.10 The pathways from the cerebellum that control balance by adjusting the body's skeletal muscles (see also Figure 6.3). LMN, lower motor neurone.

and control the fine co-ordination of voluntary movement at an unconscious level. For example, the cerebellum smoothes out muscle activity that otherwise would be jerky and erratic, especially fast movements, and it determines the extent and timing of muscle fibre contractions. In this respect it also has some influence *increasing* muscle tone, providing a balance to the muscle tone function of the basal ganglia (see p. 198). It also learns and perfects the skills of **synergy**. Synergistic skills involve the ability to co-ordinate muscle activity in relation to a moving object, using visual information from the visual cortex of the cerebrum to plot the direction and speed of the moving object. It works out the muscle response required to allow the chosen part (e.g. hand or foot) to intercept with that object, like returning a ball over the net in tennis. It means predicting ahead, since it takes time to move a limb to a new position, during which the object itself has moved. Children are born without these skills, and both synergistic skills and balance are learnt and practised from an early age. They are then pre-programmed (like many other motor skills) and function with very little or no conscious thought. A Wimbledon tennis champion must spend many hours teaching the cerebellum that particular synergistic skill. Since visual information is crucial for this function, the cerebellum has some influence and control over eyeball movements, vital in tracking moving objects.

Reflexes

Various **reflexes** exist to provide stability during movement and fast responses to adverse stimuli and are a safeguard against falling and injury. A reflex consists of a sensory input to the brain or cord, an integration or control centre, and a motor output to the relevant muscle group, i.e. the components of a **reflex arc** (Figure 9.11). Painful sensory impulses pass into the posterior spinal cord and cross to the front on the same side via a **connector** (or **association**) neurone to the cell body of an LMN. The impulses from this LMN pass out of the cord to the muscle, which then contracts to pull the limb away from the source of the pain. **Deep tendon** (or **stretch extensor**) reflexes include the **patella reflex**, where the patella tendon is tapped below the patella bone with a clinical hammer. The **knee jerk** that follows is caused first by stretching the sensory **muscle spindle** within the thigh muscle with the hammer tap, thus sending impulses into the cord. This then activates the LMN at the same level as the sensory input, and motor impulses are sent back to the same muscle making it contract slightly (to correct

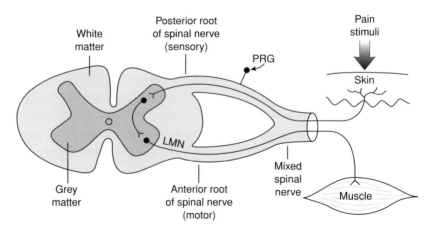

FIGURE 9.11 The reflex arc. A special sensory neurone takes painful impulses from the periphery to the cord. Impulses pass to the brain, but at the same time interneurones cross the cord from the posterior sensory to the anterior motor areas of the grey matter, and the lower motor neurone conveys an impulse to the muscles to move the part from harm. LMR, lower motor neurone; PRG, posterior root ganglion.

the original stretch). The **flexor** (or **withdrawal**) **response** is created by the application of painful stimuli to a limb, causing pain stimuli to pass into the cord. Again an LMN fires in response to contract the flexor muscles of that same limb while relaxing the extensor muscles. At the same time, the impulse crosses the midline in the cord and causes the opposite response in the other limb, which then extends (called the **crossed extensor response**) (Figure 9.12).

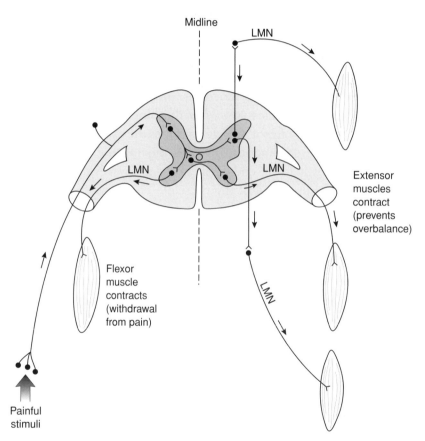

Midline

LMN

LMN

LMN

Extensor
muscles
contract
(prevents
overbalance)

Flexor
muscle
contracts
(withdrawal
from pain)

LMN

Painful
stimuli

FIGURE 9.12 The cross reflex. Painful stimuli affecting one side of the body causes flexion of the muscles on that side via the reflex arc (Figure 9.11) in order to withdraw from the pain. At the same time impulses cross to the other side and stimulate extensor muscles at several levels above and below the level affected to prevent overbalancing.

The muscles

The **end organ** of any motor system is the **muscle**, a specialist tissue with the sole function of contraction. Muscles are of three types: **skeletal muscle**, which is attached to the bones and serves to allow *voluntary* movement; **smooth muscle**, which forms the walls of internal *tubes*, such as blood vessels and the digestive tract, and is *involuntary*; and **cardiac muscle** in the heart wall, which contracts *involuntary*. Muscle is the only tissue in the body that can itself move; anything else that moves, like bones or blood, is moved by a muscle. Muscles *pull*, but cannot *push*; but smooth muscle constructed in a ring or around a tube wall can constrict to close the ring or tube lumen, e.g. a **sphincter** or the wall of the bronchus. In the limbs, skeletal muscles are set in opposing positions around joints, **antagonistic pairs**, so called because these muscles have opposing functions: one muscle to *bend* the joint (the **flexor**), and one muscle to *straighten* the joint (the **extensor**) (Figure 9.13). Contracting the flexor muscle stretches the extensor muscle, and vice versa. Muscle contraction involves moving the **insertion** (the *travelling* and mostly lower end of the muscle) towards the **origin** (the *fixed* and mostly upper end of the muscle). The nerve innervation of the various types of muscle are different: the skeletal muscle is *controlled* by the pyramidal and extra-pyramidal tract systems, the smooth muscle is *controlled* by the **autonomic nervous system** (**ANS**) and the cardiac

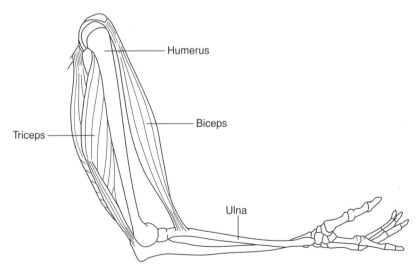

Figure 9.13 Antagonistic muscle pairs. In this example the flexor is the biceps and the extensor is the triceps muscles of the upper arm.

muscle is *regulated* by the ANS. Between the nerve and the *voluntary skeletal muscle* is the **neuromuscular junction**, a gap where a neurotransmitter called **acetylcholine** is active in passing the impulse from the neurone to the muscle cells.

Movement observations

Disorders of movement can be classified by the system that is causing the problem, i.e. pyramidal or extra-pyramidal tract disorders, basal ganglia or cerebellar disorders, or diseases of the muscles themselves. Nurses can contribute significantly to the understanding of the patient's problem, identifying the patient's needs and necessary medical interventions by observing abnormalities of movement.

Observations of movement are best achieved in conscious patients, either by watching as patients attempt movement or by requesting patients to undergo specific movements for the purpose of observation. Walking is a good opportunity to observe a patient's ability to move, whereby different forms of gait, i.e. the manner an individual walks, may be seen and balance can be assessed. Loss of consciousness removes all such *purposeful* movements and would probably mean that any movements observed are spontaneous and reflex-type activities.

Neurological assessment of the motor systems is usually carried out by specialist doctors or nurses who work in neuromedical or neurosurgical units (see Hickey 1997). However, all nurses should be able to identify gross abnormalities of movement in many care settings: in particular the accident and emergency or trauma unit, establishments caring for elderly people and outpatients' departments. The basic questions to establish are:

1 Can the patient walk properly, or are there noticeable difficulties with mobility, like dragging one foot or being unable to balance?
2 Can the patient talk properly, or are there noticeable problems with speech, like slurring of words?
3 Does the patient show any abnormal movements, like shaking or inability to sit still?

We are all familiar with the normal and expected range and types of movement, which is why abnormalities of movement tend to become quite obvious as patients make efforts to get around and communicate.

Movement problems could be classified into *losses* and *excesses*. Losses include a reduced level of movement, called **hypokinesia** (kinetics = movement, hypo = lower than normal level), the inability to *initiate* a movement, like being unable to start to walk, called **akinesia** (the letter *a* before a word means without), and a total loss of movement, referred to as a **paralysis**. **Paresis** is a weakness of muscle movement and is a condition similar to, but less severe than, paralysis. Excesses include **dyskinesia** (abnormal movements), **hyperkinesia** (an increase in involuntary movement, like tremor, an uncontrolled shaking of limbs) and **akathisia** (motor restlessness that prevents the individual from sitting down).

Movement losses

Paralysis and weakness

A total loss of the ability to move is paralysis, a major neurological deficit that may be local (e.g. in one limb) or involve wider aspects of the nervous system. **Hemiplegia**, a paralysis of either the left or right side of the body, affects those suffering from a **cerebrovascular accident** (**CVA**, or **stroke**) to various degrees. CVAs are bleeds into the brain, or an obstruction to the blood supply to the brain, resulting in brain damage. This very often involves the motor cortex and the major pathways from this area, the pyramidal tracts. Since these tracts mostly cross in the medulla (see p. 194), a *left* hemiplegia indicates a stroke on the *right* side of the brain, and vice versa. The degree of movement loss depends on the extent of the bleed and its location within the brain. Small bleeds close to the brain surface may only result in *weakness* on one side, called a **hemiparesis**, with good prospects for some recovery, whereas larger or deeper bleeds may cause profound paralysis with some permanent deficit. A CVA is an example of a UMN lesion leading to **spastic paralysis** in the longer term, where *spastic* means the stiffening and contracture of the muscles of the affected limbs if inadequate preventative measures are taken. The arm is held in a bent (= **flexed**) position and the spastic hemiparesis creates a characteristic gait where the leg *circles* stiffly outwards then inwards with a pointed toe while walking.

Unlike hemiplegia, **paraplegia** results in the loss of function of the lower limbs, and mobility usually requires a wheelchair. Paraplegia is often associated with spinal injuries where the cord is damaged, severing the pyramidal motor tracts (MI and MII) at a point in the thoracic or lumbar regions. Such trauma cuts of any opportunity for the brain to control the muscles below the level of the injury. A similar injury higher in the spine, the cervical region, may include a loss of movement below this level, i.e. a tetraplegia, involving all four limbs and the trunk. Another cause of lower limb paralysis is **poliomyelitis**, an infectious disease that damages the cell body of the LMNs or their axons passing from the cord. LMN lesions result in a **flaccid paralysis**, where muscles of the paralysed limbs become loose and floppy (loss of muscle tone) with complete loss of reflexes, and **foot drop** (a failure of the muscles that retain the foot at the normal right angle to the leg).

The loss of the ability to perform *purposeful* movements is **apraxia** (a = without, praxia = performing movements), i.e. movements are possible but meaningless. The problem is *not* caused by simple paralysis or weakness, nor is it due to a lack of comprehension or motivation. It may be the result of a lesion in the parietal association cortex (see p. 192) along with disturbance to sensory interpretation and integration. Different forms of apraxia may occur and depend on which side of the brain is affected (see p. 140). **Dyspraxia** (dys = difficulty; praxia = performing movements) is the difficulty in carrying out skilled movements with no evidence of disorder of the primary motor pathways. This is *not* the same as paralysis, which usually *does* involve the primary motor pathways. Apraxia and dyspraxia are functional developmental disorders of differing severity: apraxia is a total loss of purposeful movements and dyspraxia is a difficulty in carrying out skilled purposeful movements. Both disorders disturb the development of different systems, e.g. **verbal dyspraxia** (speech difficulty and delay), or **motor dyspraxia** (difficulty with body movement co-ordination, including balance and walking); a child with **motor dyspraxia** may be called a *clumsy child*.

Another motor problem is **multiple sclerosis (MS)**, an **autoimmune disease** of the neuronal myelin sheath, which breaks down and is replaced by scar tissue (a **demyelination** disease). Autoimmune diseases occur when the body's immune system identifies part of the body as foreign (or *alien*) tissue and begins to destroy it. The reason is not fully known but currently viral infections of the affected tissues are suspected. MS can affect any neurone, motor and sensory, and it causes a wide range of symptoms of varying degrees that can pass from *remissions* (periods of no or few symptoms) to *relapses* (periods of worse symptoms). Those signs affecting movement include spastic limb weakness with exaggerated reflexes (UMN pyramidal signs) and an ataxia (a cerebellar sign, see p. 211).

Motor neurone disease (**MND**) is another progressive degeneration of neurones, this time the pyramidal (corticospinal) tract fibres, some cranial nerve nuclei and some LMNs within the cord. It causes severe movement losses involving motor control of the swallow reflex, and death occurs within a few years. The usual age of onset is 40–60 years; the cause is unknown and there is no treatment available. Three different aspects characterise this disease: (1) **progressive muscular atrophy** (**PMA**), (2) **progressive bulbar palsy** (**PBP**) and (3) **amyotrophic lateral sclerosis** (**ALS**). Patients with this disorder will first develop one of these three aspects, which will then remain dominant. Most patients will eventually show signs of all three to varying degrees. Those in whom PMA is dominant have the least severe form and can have a survival rate of up to 15 years or more. PBP causes deterioration of parts of the brain stem, and it has the worst symptoms and the shortest life expectancy. It causes deterioration of swallowing, with choking on food, and muscle paralysis of the tongue and throat. ALS is a progressive combination of **amyotrophy**, i.e. muscle wasting caused by a loss of LMNs, and **lateral sclerosis**, a loss of UMNs in the corticospinal tracts of the spinal cord. The main features are muscular weakness and **atrophy** (= wasting of muscles), with **fasciculation** (= twitching of muscles) in two or more limbs. The intellect and sensory systems are completely unaffected and remain intact throughout.

Muscular diseases also cause weakness and paralysis. **Myasthenia gravis** is a disorder of the neuromuscular junction: acetylcholine (see p. 205) cannot bind to the receptors properly and muscle cells are unable to sustain repeated contraction during exercise so that they fatigue quickly. The receptors are blocked by antibodies, plus there is a reduced amount of acetylcholine available at the synapse. The **thymus gland**, part of the lymphatic and immune systems in the chest may be the site of production of the antibodies concerned and removal of this gland, plus drugs to improve acetylcholine function are options for treatment. The various **muscular dystrophies** form a group of disabling diseases involving the muscle itself. Several of these disorders are genetically inherited, like **Duchenne's muscular dystrophy** (DMD). This disease is the commonest in the group and affects mostly boys, although the gene involved is carried by females. Fat infiltrates the main muscles during childhood leading to deterioration in walking and other movement, with complete mobility loss by the time of adolescence.

Life expectancy may only be 20–29 years. **Myopathies** (myo = muscle, path = disease) is the term used to describe a failure of muscle development with weakness, muscle pain and cramps early in life, again often due to genetic inheritance. The weakness may be severe and cause major mobility difficulties that can be progressive throughout life.

Increased muscle tone (rigidity)

Disturbances to basal ganglia function, as in **Parkinson's disease**, can cause an increase in muscle tone, known as **hypertonia**; muscles become rigid and fail to allow full body movement. In Parkinson's disease the limbs are severely limited in function; the legs in particular create a shuffling gait and sufferers cannot lift their feet properly. The body takes on a forward stance and often moves faster than the feet can; patients may therefore lose their balance and fall. Nurses observing these patients should be aware of the potential for injury. The muscle tone increase is due to the failure of the basal ganglia's role of inhibiting excess muscle tone; an excess that is therefore passed onto the muscle. James Parkinson, a Shoreditch general practitioner, described the condition as *paralysis agitans* (i.e. agitated paralysis), which neatly describes the two main features: rigidity and tremor. Parkinson's disease is progressive due to the relentless destruction of the substantia nigra, with a corresponding gradual loss of the neurotransmitter dopamine in the substantia nigra to corpus striatum pathway. The reason for the loss of cells in the substantia nigra is unknown and untreatable, and will eventually lead to the patient's death. It would appear that the symptoms do not occur until the dopamine loss reaches 80%, indicating the **asymptomatic** (= without symptoms) onset of this disease which is very gradual over a number of years. On average, the age that symptoms become obvious is about 60 years or more, but the process leading to those symptoms must have started earlier in life. Treatment is aimed at the replacement of the dopamine in this part of the brain, effectively reducing the symptoms, particularly the rigidity, and therefore improving the quality of life.

Other forms of rigidity are **decortication**, an *abnormal flexion response*, and **decerebration**, an *abnormal extensor response* of the limbs (Figure 9.14). The symptoms of these disorders and their causes are shown in Table 9.1.

Adduction is movement of a limb *towards* the midline of the body, i.e. held against the side of the body; **internal rotation** is a twisting of

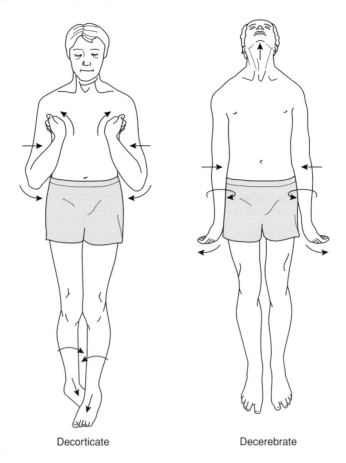

Decorticate   Decerebrate

FIGURE 9.14 Decorticate and decerebrate symptoms. In decorticate symptoms the elbows, wrists and fingers are flexed with adduction of the arms, the legs are inwardly rotated and the feet are plantar flexed. In decerebrate symptoms the head is extended with the jaws clenched shut, the arms are adducted with stiffly extended elbows, the forearms are hyperpronated and the wrists and fingers are flexed, the legs are stiffly extended and the feet are plantar flexed.

the limb *inwards*; **pronation** is a *palm downwards* position of the forearm and hand (Figure 9.14). **Plantar flexion** is a downward movement of the foot; the toes point away from the body at an angle of as much as 45° from the normal right-angle position of the foot. Decerebrate symptoms can be severe enough to include stiff clenching of the jaw, neck extension and arching of the back.

TABLE 9.1 The symptoms and causes of decortication and decerebration

Rigidity	Arms	Legs	Cause
Decortication	Hyperflexion of each of the joints with adduction of the limb	Extension of legs with internal rotation and plantar flexion of foot	A high cerebral lesion interrupting the corticospinal (pyramidal) tracts
Decerebration	Elbow extension, wrist flexion with limb adduction and pronated forearms	Stiff extension of legs with plantar flexion of foot	A hypothalamic or thalamic lesion involving the brain stem

Ataxia

Ataxia is a difficult and abnormal gait, or walking, with specific forms of ataxia indicating particular neuromuscular disorders. The gait of spastic hemiparesis seen in CVA and the shuffling gait of Parkinson's disease have both been described (see p. 206 and p. 209). **Cerebellar ataxia** is caused by a disorder of the cerebellum or its tracts. It produces an unsteady staggering gait with difficulty on turning and balance loss when the feet come together, so the feet are held apart. **Sensory ataxia** is an unsteady gait, again with feet wide apart. During walking each leg is lifted high followed by the foot being *slapped* on the floor. Since the patient is unable to feel the floor because of absent sensory feedback, it becomes necessary for the patient to watch the ground to ensure his foot is safely in contact before putting any weight on it. This is due to a destruction of the somatic sensory pathways of the spinal cord, as in **tabes dorsalis**, a spinal cord complication of the infectious disease **syphilis**. **Scissor gait** is caused by a bilateral spastic weakness of the leg muscles. The legs are moved slowly forwards over short steps; the thighs tend to cross over each other in turn.

Movement excesses

Tremor

The shaking seen in the limbs in Parkinson's disease comes in two forms: a *course* tremor noticed in the whole limb, and a *fine* tremor found in the hands and fingers. This fine tremor has been called *pill-rolling*, since this is the action taken during the manual production of pills before mechanisation. Parkinson's tremor disappears as the limbs are put into conscious motion, but returns at rest. Tremor is a very noticeable symptom and is very destructive to the patient's confidence, motor activities and natural behaviour patterns.

Athetosis, chorea and ballism

Huntington's disease is a genetically inherited disorder caused by a gene mutation on the fourth chromosome (Bentley 1999). It results in a progressive degeneration of the corpus striatum of the basal ganglia, with cell losses in the frontal and parietal lobes of the cerebral cortex. Unwanted involuntary movements are a characteristic of this disease, and these are **athetosis** (slow writhing movements of the limbs, face and tongue) and **chorea** (fast twitching of whole limbs and body). If these two movements occur together the words are combined, i.e. **choreoathetosis**. The major distinctions between them are the speed (*sudden* chorea movements compared with the *slow* athetosis movements) and the nature of the movement (in chorea *jerky* and *twitching* movements that are not repeated; in athetosis *writhing* movements). Observers will note that the patient appears to be unable to sit still. Chorea can sometimes occur in children (**Sydenham's chorea**), often as a result of **rheumatic fever**, caused mostly by an immune response to the bacterium *Streptococcus*. The child or adolescent shows sudden, irregular and uncontrolled movements of no real purpose, but unlike Huntington's disease this is not a permanent problem.

Uncontrolled violent movements of a whole limb, involving flinging the arm suddenly in any direction, is called **ballism**. The appearance of this phenomenon may be sudden and frightening. **Monoballism** is the term used if a single limb only is involved, and **hemiballism** indicates that both limbs on one side are affected. The violent nature of this movement is due to the involvement of the **subthalamic nucleus** in the lesion.

The immobile patient

Immobility removes the patient's ability to sustain the very basic needs of life, and these must be provided by the nurse. But practical care alone is not enough, the nurse's observations of the immobile patient are critical to the patient's progress:

1 Observation of the skin is vital for:
   (a) assessing any dehydration, i.e. when the skin is dry and can be pulled into folds which remain when released. Dehydration is a severe lack of fluids in the tissues, both the **intracellular** (intra = inside, cellular = the cells) and the **extracellular** (extra = outside, cellular = the cells, or **tissue fluid**) fluids;
   (b) preventing **decubitus ulcers** (= pressure sores), caused both by constricted blood supply to the tissues when compressed by body weight and by friction eroding the surface of the skin when the patient is moved. Assessment of a patient's risk of skin breakdown is often made using the **Waterlow scale** (Waterlow 1992) or the **Norton scale** (Alexander *et al.* 1994).
   (c) maintaining personal cleanliness.
2 Observing the mouth is vital for:
   (a) preventing dehydration, causing a dry mouth with poor saliva production;
   (b) preventing infections, causing red, swollen gums and halitosis (foul-smelling breath), pain and difficulty with eating and the risk of complications, like throat, chest, ear and brain infections.
3 Observing the urine is vital for:
   (a) assessing the output to maintain fluid balance and reduce the risk of renal disorders (see Chapter 5);
   (b) preventing urinary tract infections (see Chapter 5).
4 Observing the bowel function is vital for:
   (a) assessing the output, to prevent constipation or diarrhoea (see Chapter 6).
5 Observing the level of consciousness is vital for:
   (a) prevention of confusion or coma (see Chapter 7).
6 Observing the respirations is vital for:
   (a) maintaining adequate ventilation and oxygenation (see Chapter 4);
   (b) preventing chest infections (see Chapter 4).
7 Observing body temperature is vital for:
   (a) assessing the patient's ability to control body temperature (see Chapter 1);
   (b) preventing or detecting any underlying infections.
8 Observing the ability to communicate is vital for:
   (a) assessment of mental function, especially mood, which may be depressed;
   (b) assessment of problems like pain.
9 Observing the ability to eat and drink is vital for:
   (a) assessing the patient's nutritional status (see chapter 6);
   (b) preventing hunger, dehydration and hospital-acquired malnutrition.

10 Observing the sleep cycle pattern is vital for:

   (a) assessing that the patient has enough rest.

11 Observing the pattern of mobility possible, in each limb and joint is vital for:

   (a) assessing what mobility the patient can achieve and maximising this (see this chapter);

   (b) assessing what mobility assistance the patient will need in terms of professional help, such as physiotherapy, and mobility aids, such as a wheelchair.

With modern technology available, and given what is known about the complications of bed rest, immobility must *not* mean a lifetime confined to bed.

Key points

- Pre-programming of movement is the essence of the learning process and allows movement to occur at a subconscious level.
- The motor cortex cells are arranged in a manner that reflects the basic body plan.
- The pyramidal tracts descend from the motor cortex.
- The pyramidal system is two-neuronal, consisting of an upper motor neurone (UMN) from brain to cord and a lower motor neurone (LMN) from cord to muscle.
- The parietal association cortex integrates sensory stimuli necessary for voluntary movement.
- The extra-pyramidal system controls voluntary movement at a subconscious level.
- The basal ganglia have a role in controlling slow, sustained movements and in maintaining muscle tone.
- Muscle tone is a state of tension of the muscle essential for contraction.
- The cerebellum is important for balance, posture, smoothing out muscle movements and synergistic skills, i.e. the ability to match muscle activity to a moving object.
- Reflexes provide stability during movement and fast responses to adverse stimuli. A reflex arc has a sensory input to the cord, a control centre and a motor output to the muscle.
- Muscles are of three types: skeletal muscle attached to bones, allowing voluntary movement, smooth muscle forming walls of internal tubes, allowing involuntary movement and cardiac muscle in the heart wall.

- The various types of muscle have different nerve innervation: skeletal muscle is controlled by the pyramidal and extra-pyramidal systems, smooth muscle is controlled by the autonomic nervous system, and cardiac muscle is regulated by the autonomic nervous system.
- Paralysis is a loss of movement: hemiplegia is paralysis of either the left or right half of the body, paraplegia is paralysis of the lower half of the body and tetraplegia is paralysis of the body from the neck down.
- Cerebrovascular accident (CVA) or stroke is a bleed into the brain or an obstruction of the blood supply to the brain.
- Poliomyelitis is an infectious disease that damages the cell body of the lower motor neurone.
- Multiple sclerosis is an autoimmune disease of the myelin sheath, which breaks down and is replaced by scar tissue.
- Myasthenia gravis is the inability of acetylcholine to bind at the neuromuscular junction, which causes the muscles to be unable to sustain repeated contraction.
- Muscular dystrophies are often genetically inherited. Duchenne's muscular dystrophy affects mostly boys. Fat accumulates in the main muscles during childhood, leading to deterioration of walking with complete mobility loss by the time of adolescence.
- Parkinson's disease is a degeneration of the basal ganglia, causing an increase in muscle tone resulting in rigidity and tremor.
- Decortication is an abnormal flexion response caused by a high cerebral lesion interrupting the corticospinal (pyramidal) tracts. Decerebration is an abnormal extensor response caused by a hypothalamic or thalamic lesion involving the brain stem.
- Ataxia is difficult or abnormal gait (method of walking).
- Motor neurone disease is a progressive degeneration of neurones of the pyramidal and bulbar tracts.
- Huntington's disease is a genetically inherited disorder resulting in a progressive degeneration of the corpus striatum with cell losses in the frontal and parietal lobes.
- Unwanted involuntary movements are called chorea (sudden and jerky movements) and athetosis (slow writhing movements).

References

Alexander M., Fawcett J. and Runciman P. (eds) (1994) *Nursing Practice, Hospital and Home: The Adult*. Churchill Livingston, London.
Bentley P. (1999) Dementia demystified. *Nursing Times* 95(45): 47–49.

Hickey J. V. (1997) *The Clinical Practice of Neurological and Neurosurgical Nursing*, 4th edn., Lippincott, Philadelphia.

Pinel J. P. J. (1993) *Biopsychology*, 2nd edn. Allyn and Bacon.

Waterlow J. (1992) A policy that protects: the Waterlow pressure sore prevention/treatment policy, in Horne E. and Cowan T. (eds) *Staff Nurse's Survival Guide*, 2nd edn. Wolfe Publishing, London.

Index